THE MINDFUL FREAK-OUT

Also by Eric Goodman

Your Anxiety Beast and You: A compassionate guide to living in an increasingly anxious world
By integrating therapeutic methods from compassion-focused therapy, cognitive behavioural therapy, and Acceptance and Commitment Therapy, this book takes you through step-by-step strategies to cope with the howling of anxiety in your mind and the physical effects of anxiety on your body. It then focuses on ways to come up with 'teachable moments', so your anxiety can learn that what you fear is not actually a threat.

Social Courage: Coping and thriving with the reality of social anxiety
This book presents a step-by-step approach and structured program for minimizing suffering in the face of social anxiety while giving you the tools to boldly go towards your social goals. Whether you are struggling with social anxiety of phobic proportions or are just held back when it comes to public speaking or meeting a specific social goal, this book presents your path forward.

THE
MINDFUL
FREAK-OUT

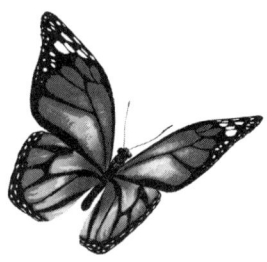

A rescue manual for being at your best
when life is at its worst

ERIC GOODMAN Ph.D.

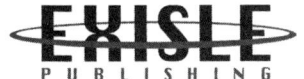

First published 2024

Exisle Publishing Pty Ltd
PO Box 864, Chatswood, NSW 2057, Australia
226 High Street, Dunedin, 9016, New Zealand
www.exislepublishing.com

Copyright © 2024 in text: Eric Goodman

Eric Goodman asserts the moral right to be identified as the author of this work.

All rights reserved. Except for short extracts for the purpose of review, no part of this book may be reproduced, stored in a retrieval system or transmitted in any form or by any means, whether electronic, mechanical, photocopying, recording or otherwise, without prior written permission from the publisher.

A CiP record for this book is available from the National Library of Australia.

ISBN 978-1-922539-36-6

Designed by Mark Thacker
Typeset in 11.5 on 17.25 Minion Pro Regular
Printed by Sheridan

This book uses paper sourced under ISO 14001 guidelines from well-managed forests and other controlled sources.

10 9 8 7 6 5 4 3 2 1

Disclaimer

This book is a general guide only and should never be a substitute for the skill, knowledge and experience of a qualified health professional dealing with the facts, circumstances and symptoms of a particular case. The information presented in this book is based on the research, training and professional experience of the author, and is true and complete to the best of their knowledge. However, this book is intended only as an informative guide; it is not intended to replace or countermand the advice given by the reader's health provider. Because each person and situation is unique, the author and the publisher urge the reader to check with a qualified health professional before using any procedure where there is a question as to its appropriateness. The author, publisher and their distributors are not responsible for any adverse effects or consequences resulting from the use of the information in this book. It is the responsibility of the reader to consult a physician or other qualified healthcare professional regarding their personal care. The intent of the information provided is to be helpful; however, there is no guarantee of results associated with the information provided.

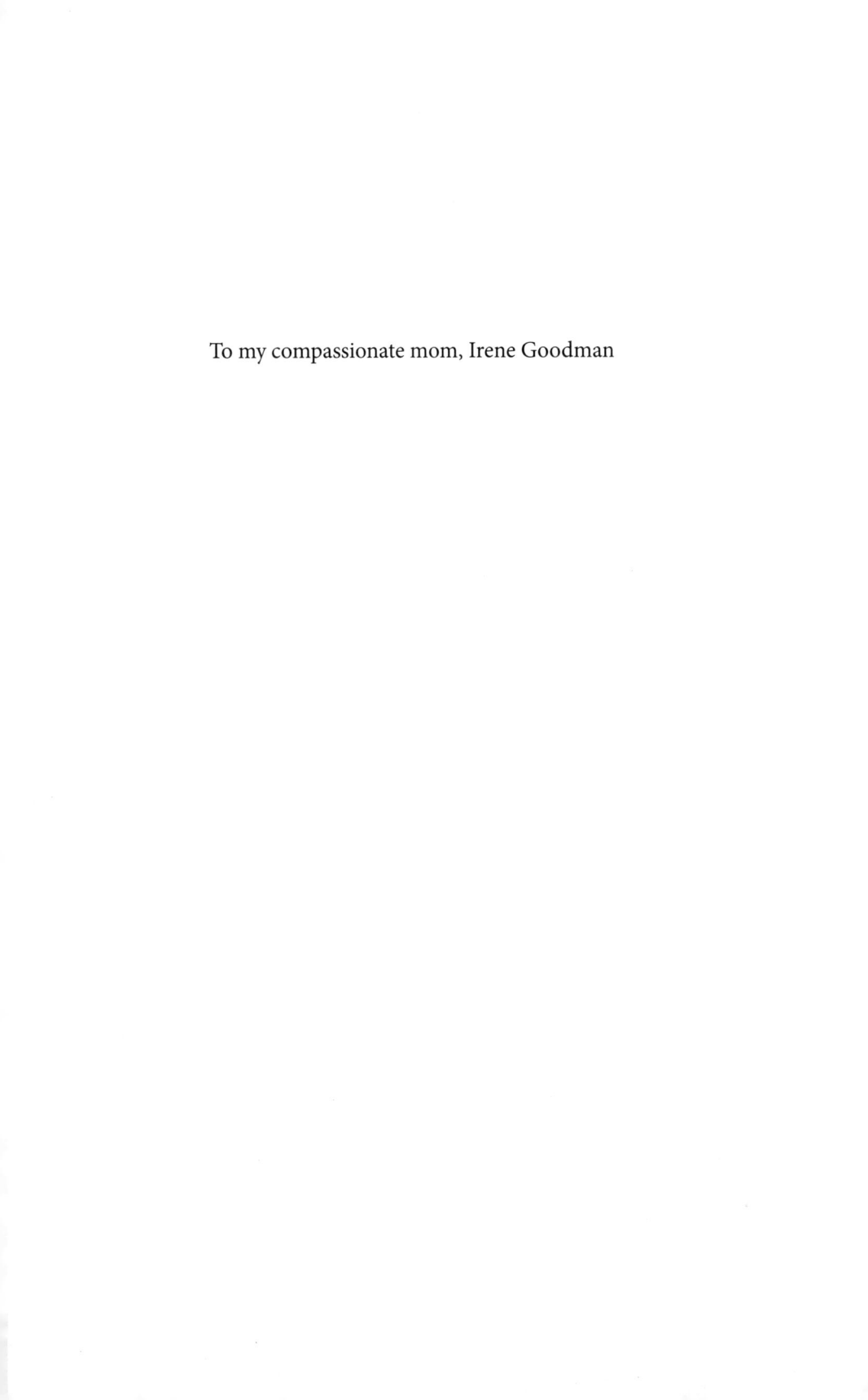

To my compassionate mom, Irene Goodman

Contents

How to use this book *1*

Quick-start guide for responding to highly distressing moments *3*

Introduction *9*

PART 1:
Getting off emotional autopilot (compassionate awareness)

1. When your emotions hijack you *23*
2. Notice suffering and slowing down *27*
3. Setting an intention to do what is helpful *31*
4. Anchoring your attention in the present moment *39*

PART 2:
Facing painful moments with compassion (compassionate acceptance)

5. The problem with fighting your feelings *61*
6. Engaging your compassionate mind *69*
7. Compassionate mind training *95*
8. Noticing and releasing struggle *115*
9. Unhooking from unhelpful thoughts *123*

PART 3:
Responding based on your Best Self (compassionate action)

10. Noticing and naming urges *141*
11. Choosing your Best Self response *149*
12. Committing to taking action and noticing the outcome *173*
13. Navigating common freak-outs *191*

PART 4:
Overcoming challenges to acting with compassion

14. Fears, blocks and resistances to compassion *223*
15. When things don't go well: compassionate self-correction vs punishing self-criticism *233*

Beyond freaking out *243*

Appendix 1: The emotionally distressing moment rescue exercise *245*
Appendix 2: Exercise record form *250*
Appendix 3: Rescue strategy for being at your best when life is at its worst: brief outline *255*

Acknowledgements *257*
Endnotes *259*
Index *265*

How to use this book

This book was written as a guide for people who are experiencing suffering during moments of emotional pain, for example:

- when a panic attack strikes!
- coming face to face with something you find terrifying (being in the social spotlight or experiencing heavy turbulence on a flight)!
- wrestling with insomnia, yet again!
- being tormented by your own thoughts!
- losing your temper and acting in a way you later regret!
- feeling overwhelmed by despair — like you just can't take it anymore!
- when life hands you a very unwelcome surprise (death of a loved one, serious illness, job or relationship loss)!

During such moments, distressing emotions can take over and lead you to act in ways that actually multiply your suffering. And it may drive you to behave in ways that you later regret.

This book was written to be a guide for navigating life's difficult moments in a way that minimizes suffering while maximizing values-based responding.

The book comes with a quick-start guide (just like you might find when you buy a phone or printer) so you can begin to take effective action right away to address your suffering. The quick-start guide breaks down key evidence-based strategies into concise steps so they can be of immediate use.

Then, reading beyond the quick-start guide, you will strengthen your understanding of how to apply these concepts during your most emotionally painful moments. The exercises in this book are designed to increase your ability to respond to emotionally challenging moments in ways that reduce your suffering while increasing values-based responding — rather than impulsive, emotion-driven reacting.

You might notice that some strategies in this book come easily for you while others may take time and practice to more fully develop. For example, you might find that you are good with mindful awareness, but compassion is more challenging for you to develop. This book is filled with exercises designed to build your skills in areas that don't come easily to you.

Quick-start guide for responding to highly distressing moments

Here are evidence-based steps you can take when suffering during emotionally distressing moments:

Step 1:
Get off autopilot (compassionate awareness)

Your internal threat system is designed to try to take over during 'threatening' moments and propel you to take steps to fight or flee from a threat. This is important when survival is at stake but can be unhelpful when your threat system is only misperceiving the situation to be threatening.

What helps:

THE MINDFUL FREAK-OUT

Notice suffering and slow down
You may find that your mind and body are reacting with urgency — filling you with painful fight-or-flight emotions. Notice suffering in yourself or others and step back, and stop reacting for a moment. If you are around others and it is appropriate, you can take a brief break from the interaction (perhaps take a bathroom break or get a glass of water). Allow yourself to slow down.

Set an intention to do what is helpful
Rather than impulsively reacting to the painful moment, allow your inner tone to become calm and caring as you set an intention to do something to improve the situation in a helpful way.

You might say to yourself, 'This is a difficult moment. May I do what is helpful right now.'

Anchor in the moment using breathing and senses
Your attention may get pulled to remembering the past or anticipating the future ('They should not have done that!' or 'If I make a mistake, I might be humiliated!'). Come back to now by anchoring yourself in the present moment using your five senses and breathing. Notice what you can see, hear, feel with your body, smell and taste.

You might notice that you are holding your breath or breathing shallowly. Invite your breathing to become deeper and more rhythmic. Slow down your exhalation. Give yourself a moment to just breathe.

Step 2:
Face the painful moment with compassion (compassionate acceptance)

When you are faced with painful emotions, you might be tempted to struggle with them or run from them. If you do this, however, it can intensify your suffering. At times, it may give short-term relief, but increase long-term suffering. Instead, you can choose to turn and face painful emotions while taking steps to ease your suffering.

What helps:

Engage your compassionate mind
Meeting your distress with compassion can help balance out your threat system, decrease suffering, and put you in a mindset that increases your ability to respond to this difficult moment using your values as a guide rather than reacting based on emotion.

One way to do this is to try to recall a time when you were at your compassionate best, for example when helping a friend or family member who was suffering. Try to recall the feeling of having a sense of inner strength, wisdom to not judge them, and how you were focused on being warm, kind and helpful. Try to get a sense of those qualities (even a little) right now. Like an actor getting absorbed into their character, take on the role of your compassionate ideal self.

If your distress involves other people, try recalling that everyone struggles and suffers at times — that human life can be very difficult. Just like all of us, this other person is doing their best based on their genes, their upbringing, and things that have happened to them that they did not choose.

THE MINDFUL FREAK-OUT

Notice and release struggle

Fighting to get rid of your painful emotions can make them more intense, increase your suffering, and further teach your threat system that you are in 'danger'.

For this moment, see if you can notice where you are automatically struggling against your painful emotions. See if you can let go of struggle and allow the feelings to sit softly in your feet, legs, stomach, back, hands, arms, chest, neck, jaw, and around your eyes and forehead. Focus on increasing your willingness to compassionately face the emotions that have shown up for you — without struggle.

Unhook from unhelpful thoughts

Your mind may be hooking onto threat-thoughts that are not helpful for you such as: 'I must get rid of this unpleasant feeling right now! I can't do this!', 'If I fail at this, I will be a failure!', 'I'll feel this way forever!', 'Feelings like these are dangerous!' or 'I must win this argument!'

Remember that you are not your thoughts, nor are you responsible for the 'mind-noise' your brain automatically generates. See if you can unhook from the unhelpful thoughts. Watch them come and go without grabbing onto them or pushing them away. You can treat them like ocean waves, coming and going with you watching from the shore rather than diving in and being carried away by them.

Step 3: Respond based on your 'Best Self' (compassionate action)

The goal of this step is to choose and implement an action (or strategic inaction) that is consistent with who you want to be. A Best Self action

Quick-start guide for responding to highly distressing moments

is values-based and seeks to ease your suffering in the long term, even if it means making a less comfortable choice right now. For example, choosing to go to a dinner party even though you feel socially anxious, because it can lead to a valued goal such as friendship. Facing a fear can also ease your suffering over time, though it might be uncomfortable initially.

What helps:

Notice and name your urge to react

Your threat emotions will come with automatic urges to react to difficult moments in specific ways. For example, having the urge to call the dinner party host and cancel because you are nervous. You reclaim some power over your threat system by noticing and naming the urge or instinct that you have right now ('I am aware of the urge to avoid going to the dinner party').

Choose your Best Self response

Imagine that you are the best version of yourself. From that mindset, notice whether acting on your emotion-driven urges would be consistent with that best version of you. If not, how would you choose to respond to this difficult moment? Another question you could ask yourself is what would you advise someone you care deeply about to do in this situation?

Act and notice the outcome

Now is the moment of choice. You can choose to move towards being the person you want to be, or you can move away. Over time you can notice whether your action (or strategic inaction) did, in fact, move you closer to values-based living. You can also notice whether it led to less suffering in the long term, even if it meant initially facing your distressing emotions.

Introduction

While working on this book, I receive a text that is the stuff of nightmares for parents: 'We have an emergency with your daughter, please give me a call!' I frantically make the call and am told that our daughter is in an ambulance on the way to a trauma centre.

Everybody freaks out sometimes

What does it mean to 'freak out?' This odd expression is something people use in a variety of contexts.

- 'When I found out she was texting with her ex, I freaked out and ended the relationship.' (Signifying anger and impulsivity.)
- 'There was a spider in my bed this morning and I freaked out!' (Signifying feeling highly anxious.)
- 'When they broke up with me, I freaked out, thinking my life was over! I couldn't stop crying.' (Signifying intense despair.)

THE MINDFUL FREAK-OUT

We all know intuitively what it is like to freak out, but what exactly is it? *The Merriam-Webster Dictionary* defines 'freak out' as: 'an act or instance of freaking out'.[1] Not the most helpful definition.

The next definition is given as: 'a gathering of hippies'. Great information for obscure trivia nights, but also not helpful.

Collins English Dictionary defines freak out as: 'to be or cause to be in a heightened emotional state, such as that of fear, anger, or excitement'.[2] This seems to capture the spirit of freaking out as used in today's jargon. We are going about our lives when, suddenly, our brain perceives or misperceives a threat and, instantly, powerful and painful emotions try to take over. Sometimes this doesn't end well for us. The emotions can hijack us and drive us to behave in ways that are impulsive and ultimately counterproductive:

- Freaking out about not being able to sleep leads to a battle against insomnia, which pushes sleep further away!
- Freaking out about feeling anxious leads to an internal struggle that inflames the anxiety into panic!
- Freaking out about giving a presentation in class or at work, which leads to an overwhelming urge to be perfect, which makes performance stiffer, awkward and painful!
- Freaking out about a big decision, which leads to endless rumination agony!
- Freaking out about something your romantic partner said or did, which leads to a big fight and, later, regret!
- Freaking out about any number of frightening things (e.g. spiders, public speaking, dating, adventure, career

opportunities), which leads to avoiding situations in life that are important to you!

Our daughter had been out of town with her track team for a competition. She had leapt over a hurdle during a race and when she landed, her femur, the largest bone in her leg, snapped like a twig.

My wife and I immediately hop into the car, adrenaline surging, and take off for the nearly three-hour drive to the trauma centre where the ambulance has taken her. As we race to get there, we get a call from one of the doctors. She confirms that our daughter's leg is broken and that she will need emergency surgery right away. To make matters worse, she says she is 'very concerned' because they can't detect a pulse in our daughter's leg or foot.

Our emotions are intensely painful. We are freaking out!

Responding to a freak-out moment

The legal system and the cosmic relationship scrap-pile are filled with people who in a freak-out moment acted impulsively and created irreparable harm to others, their relationships or their own lives. Think about all of the cases of flight attendants being assaulted by frazzled pandemic-frustrated individuals who freaked out about wearing a mask and lashed out impulsively.

We all freak out at times — meaning we all experience sudden intense surges of painful emotions. This book teaches skills for catching yourself during highly emotionally distressing moments and taking quick, proactive steps to reduce your suffering and sense of being out of control — while increasing your ability to respond to the difficult moment in ways you won't later regret, and which might even lead to personal growth.

> *The emotional distress is intense and my mind is racing.*
>
> *The anxious part of me howls in my mind: What if she loses her leg? What if she has a concussion? What if she is in excruciating pain, alone and scared in the hospital? What if she gets Covid during this ordeal? What if she dies?*
>
> *The angry part of me then shoves the anxious part aside and looks for someone to blame: I trusted those school officials with my child! Someone was being negligent! This shouldn't have happened!*
>
> *The sad part of me is full of despair and is moaning in the background: I'm a bad parent. I couldn't protect my child. Why did this have to happen? Now that Covid's less of a concern she could have had a great end to her final year in high school — now it's lost.*
>
> *I am initially hooked by these threat-thoughts. Then I realize that I have been on autopilot, struggling and suffering with emotional pain and uncertainty.*
>
> *Wait, what do I do right now?*

A 'mindless' freak-out occurs when a highly distressing situation is met with automatic, impulsive, emotion-driven reactions. When emotions get loud and painful, people often quickly and reflexively try to get past the painful moment because their distress feels too uncomfortable to bear. They get hooked by threat-thoughts and struggle against painful feelings. They can then be swept away by the circumstances, which can lead them to react in a values-inconsistent way that can bring negative consequences for themselves and others.

Don't count on not freaking out

No matter who you are or what you have accomplished in life, you are not immune to powerful, distressing emotions. They are part of what we sign up for when we are born. Yet society sends messages that if you are not feeling calm or happy you are doing something wrong or that it is a 'disorder' to feel intense, unpleasant emotions.

In this book you will learn why we freak out at times and, more importantly, you will learn an approach for handling these moments in a way that minimizes suffering and helps you respond in a values-consistent way.

I need to get off autopilot! Where do I start? Oh yes.
Slow down. Just pause for a moment (from internal struggle, not from driving to the hospital).
I realize that I am suffering right now. With a warm, kind tone, I set an intention to be of help to myself and others during this painful time. I acknowledge that this is a very distressing moment and that any loving parent in this situation would be in emotional pain. I tell myself, 'May I do something helpful in the face of this situation and these emotions.'

THE MINDFUL FREAK-OUT

Then I focus on my breath, breathing down into my stomach and slowing the release. Just drive and breathe. Now feel how it feels to sit in my seat. I grip the steering wheel and notice the hard, bumpy texture. Now I notice the sound of the car on the road, other cars nearby, and the sound of the air-conditioning in the car. I notice that the sky is a deep blue with occasional wisps of white cloud. The plains and mountains are golden yellow – not green like where I live. I notice a range of cars, trucks and RVs dotting the road ahead.

I'm here now. In the car, in this moment only. What should I do next?

I take notice of the pain I am experiencing right now. I try to wake up my compassionate mind to marshal my inner strength. I imagine how I would talk to a good friend whose daughter is being prepped for sudden emergency surgery. I imagine having the strength to be with a friend's pain. I imagine that my voice would be gentle and reassuring. I imagine that I would be there for them without reservation. My attitude would be summarized by one question: How can I help? I would also realize that their pain is a tribute to how much they love their child. I would know that this is a type of pain that is experienced universally by humans. When we love, there is sometimes great pain. Now I imagine bringing that sense of strength, wisdom to not judge the pain, and commitment to be helpful back towards myself – and my spouse, who is equally in pain in the passenger seat next to me.

Next, I shift my attention to noticing what I feel. There's a lot going on right now. Anxiety is the loudest part, but anger and sadness are in the mix. I notice the urge to not feel these painful emotions, but I know emotional avoidance comes at a big cost.

I scan my body, looking for where I am tensing, bracing and struggling. I notice that my teeth are clenched tightly. Then I notice my arms and hands are squeezing the steering wheel much harder than they need to. My stomach is also tightening. And I notice my left foot is fidgeting in response to my emotions. I allow each of those muscles to soften as much as they are willing. I surrender any struggle against the emotions.

A better way to freak out: ACT overview

This book integrates strategies from Acceptance and Commitment Therapy (ACT) and Compassion Focused Therapy (CFT). These are evidence-based therapeutic approaches aimed at reducing human suffering while encouraging people to live their best lives.

ACT is focused on six overlapping strategies designed to encourage 'psychological flexibility'. This means consciously choosing to respond to distressing thoughts and emotions in ways that are consistent with your values, rather than responding in ways you later regret. Even though you might feel frightened, you march forward to give that talk because it is in the service of something important to you. Or you feel furious when a car cuts you off, but you resist the urge to road rage and instead opt to slow down and breathe because violence is inconsistent with who you want to be.

To be psychologically flexible during a highly distressing moment, ACT initially encourages **awareness**. These awareness strategies focus on:

THE MINDFUL FREAK-OUT

- Contacting the present moment. This involves keeping your focus in the here and now, rather than allowing autopilot to keep the focus of your attention in the past ('She shouldn't have done that!') or future ('If I have a panic attack, I'll die!').
- Engaging your observing mind (what ACT calls 'self-as-context'). This is the stable part of you that is observing the various experiences in your life without getting hooked by them. It is the part of you in the background that realizes, 'I'm upset and feel like breaking something' rather than just acting on this. Getting in touch with this part of yourself helps you to make conscious choices.

Next, ACT encourages you to face your current experience with **acceptance**, rather than struggling against your own thoughts and feelings (which increases suffering). Strategies for this include:

- Acceptance. This means surrendering the battle against uncomfortable thoughts and feelings rather than inflaming them by fighting them. It doesn't mean you don't try to solve a problem. Rather, it means accepting that in the moment your experience *is* your experience. You can accept that you are feeling anxious about a big presentation at work *while* you prepare for it.
- Defusion. Our human brains say all kinds of things. Some of it is helpful and much of it is not. Defusion involves unhooking from the unhelpful thoughts rather than fusing with them. This lets us see our thoughts

for what they are — fleeting words or images. Defusion gives us distance and perspective from the mental noise, which allows us to decline automatically following orders from our minds.

Finally, ACT encourages you to **act** based on your core values (who you want to be in life) rather than letting your thoughts, emotions and impulses choose your actions for you. This involves the following strategies:

- Values. Rather than living based on emotional whims, ACT encourages you to choose how you want to be in the world rather than being driven by emotions or instincts.
- Committed action. This involves making concrete goals, based on core values, and taking the steps needed to accomplish those goals ('When I am upset with my spouse, I will cool off a bit before talking with them. Then I will try to resolve the situation in a caring and assertive way rather than trying to "win" at all costs.').

Next I work to unhook from my painful, unhelpful thoughts. The thought, 'She may never walk again,' shows up. I imagine it written on a leaf which is floating on a stream. I try to stay out of the stream and just let it float by in its own time. The thought, 'I'm a bad father – I should have been able to protect her,' tries to hook me. I let it go; it is not helpful right now. I sit back and notice anxious, angry and sad thoughts drop into focus as leaves on a stream. I let them come and go at their own pace.

Adding CFT to ACT

Compassion Focused Therapy adds an intentional focus on bringing compassion to ourselves and others during moments of suffering in order to foster a sense of inner strength to face the moment, wisdom to not judge or blame, and the commitment to do what is helpful in easing or preventing suffering. CFT teaches people to direct compassion towards themselves, be open to compassion from others, and to direct compassion towards others. A compassionate mindset can help balance out painful emotional responses to distressing situations.[3] In other words, it can help soothe the savage freak-out.

In recent years, researchers and clinicians have been combining elements from CFT and ACT approaches.[4,5] In this book, we look at such an approach as it relates to moments of intense distress.

I am faced with the decision. Who do I want to be in this painful moment? Do I want to be one with my anxious self, which has the urge to panic and drive at a ridiculously unsafe speed? Do I want to be one with my angry self, which wants to stomp into the hospital filled with blame and acrimony? Do I want to become one with my sad self, which just feels like crawling into a hole, away from the world of people and love, and surrender to this feeling of powerlessness?

There is another choice.

I actively pivot to compassion. I pledge to let go of blaming and shaming thoughts. I'll be kind and helpful to the overworked medical staff at the trauma centre. When they are frazzled, unfriendly and unclear, I will try to be patient and remember that they have been through difficult years on the front lines of the Covid battle. And I will be a persistent advocate for our daughter and will hold her hand, stroke her hair, and let her know that we are there and we care deeply. I will carry my own pain gently and with self-compassion – with the understanding that sometimes life hurts and today is one of those days. I even feel some compassion for the painful emotions themselves. I appreciate that they want what is best for me and my family, even though they are very primitive in how they express it.

My goal for you is to learn how to call upon these evidence-based strategies to guide you through your most emotionally painful moments — minimizing your suffering and refocusing on facing the challenging moment with renewed inner strength, wisdom, and a deep commitment to responding in a values-based way, rather than in a harmful, impulsive way.

My wife and I were freaking out on that drive, then in the hospital, and at various times during the next few days – and we did what we could to be helpful to ourselves and others. I know autopilot could have driven us to acting impulsively based on emotions. Instead, we did our best to stay true to our values while using a compassionate mindset to ease our suffering. We got through it the best way we could. I'm happy to say that our daughter, after a lengthy recovery period, is doing well and running with the track team at her college.

PART 1

GETTING OFF EMOTIONAL AUTOPILOT

(Compassionate Awareness)

1

WHEN YOUR EMOTIONS HIJACK YOU

Threat-based emotions *will* try to take over!

There is no more powerful instinct than the instinct to survive. This goes way back to our prehistoric days when our ancestors learned that it paid to be cautious. When they were out hunting and gathering and they heard a noise in a bush they might have thought, 'There might be a tasty bunny in that bush,' and impulsively dove right in. Or they might have thought, 'Hold on, there might be something in that bush that is bigger and hungrier than me — with sharp teeth,' and skipped the bush and went about their scrounging elsewhere.

The reality of life is that you can miss lunch regularly, but you can be lunch only once. Therefore, it paid to err on the side of being safe rather than sorry. And because of this, our brains have been fine-tuned over millions of years to be powerful, always on, threat detection and reaction machines. When our brains perceive that there is a threat, intense emotions will try to kick you out of the driver's seat of your own life so they can take over and react quickly to the 'threat'.

This can actually be helpful — if the threat you face is real, imminent, and doesn't require complex problem-solving. If you are being chased by a hungry bear, you want your threat system to instantly focus your mind and body on only that one thing: survival. It would not be adaptive to begin fleeing the chasing bear only to stop because you realize that you need to call your mum on her birthday. You certainly would not want to stop and smell the roses or daydream about your upcoming vacation. If you are driving on the highway and the car in front of you suddenly slams on its brakes, it is beneficial that your threat system takes over and reflexively guides you to slam on the brakes too, often without giving you a moment to review and consider all your options. If someone quickly throws something heavy at your head, within your field of vision, your body will likely attempt to duck or swat it away *before* you even fully register that it has been thrown.

The problem is that the challenges we face in the modern world are often more complex and less dangerous than the daily life of our hunter-gatherer ancestors. When your brain warns you of danger when you are speaking in public, going on a blind date, running late for work, watching a scary movie or riding a roller-coaster, most likely it is absurdly over-estimating the risk of catastrophe. That's what it does.

When your emotions take over and lead you to behave in a helpful way (like running away from a charging bear) they are doing the right thing (trying to help) at the right time (you are in imminent danger). However, it is much less helpful when your primitive threat system activates your fight-flight-freeze response in ways that might take you away from being the person you'd like to be. For example, snapping and yelling at your child who accidentally spilled their milk (fight), avoiding a social invitation because your anxiety screams that you will be rejected by other people (flight), or putting off writing an essay for school because you are feeling overwhelmed by perfectionistic impulses (freeze). In those and so many other situations you may benefit from learning to override your autopilot.

When you are freaking out, the first step is to get off autopilot

When you are feeling emotionally distressed and your threat system takes over, you may behave in ways you later regret. For example, think about how productive it has been to try to resolve conflict with a family member when anger is driving you. Probably not very productive. Behaving based on strong threat-based emotions can be like a revved up bull in a china shop leading to situations like:

- starting a fight with your spouse when you value a close, warm connection
- avoiding speaking up in a work meeting due to anxiety, when you would like to advance your career.

These behaviours are probably not in your best *long-term* interests. Impulsive, emotion-driven behaviours often don't turn out well.

Taking steps to turn off your autopilot

We live in the age of autopilot. Most of us wake up in the morning and automatically click into technology and begin consuming content. Our smartphones keep us constantly distracted and entertained while the content tells us what to think and desire. We are living more and more of our lives sucked into these virtual worlds. And, in those moments when we are unplugged, we are often ruminating over something in the past ('Did I say something to offend my friend?') or our attention is propelled into the future ('What if I never find love?').

To get off autopilot and have the freedom to choose how we want to behave in the world, we must return to the only place where we can grab that freedom — the present moment, just as it is. To do this, learning and practising the following strategies helps — we will look at each of them in the following three chapters:

1. Noticing suffering and slowing down.
2. Setting an intention to do what is helpful.
3. Anchoring in the moment using breathing and senses.

KEY POINTS

- We can become swept away by our emotions.
- Threat emotions can impulsively drive us to behave in ways we later regret.
- We must get off autopilot in order to have a choice in how we respond to a freak-out moment.

2

NOTICING SUFFERING AND SLOWING DOWN

The wise sage Ferris Bueller once said, 'Life moves pretty fast. If you don't stop and look around once in a while you could miss it.' Modern life moves at a frenetic pace. On top of the near-constant digital intrusions into everyday life, we are often overly busy — rushing to or from work or class, juggling hobbies and interests with bills, meal prep, child-rearing, family obligations and so forth. It is a far cry from the less complex life of our prehistoric ancestors which roughly consisted of wake up, hunt and gather, share the bounty and each other's company, then sleep and repeat.

In our hectic and overstimulated modern lives, it can be hard to slow down and think clearly at any time, let alone when our threat systems hijack our logic and reason. When distressed, it is easy to lose the ability to make a rational decision, which can lead us to overreact based on powerful threat instincts. Someone may claim to value peace and mutual respect only to find themselves yelling at their kids or honking obscenities to the person driving in front of them.

To make matters worse, in the midst of an emotionally painful moment many of us find ourselves (often without awareness) directing harsh criticism at ourselves for making minor mistakes or being humanly imperfect. We even beat ourselves up for the feelings we experience ('I'm such a cry-baby!'). In these moments, we might say cruel things to ourselves that we would never consider directing at any other human on the planet. This can further inflame painful emotions and inner suffering.

The activation of our threat systems leads to painful and powerful emotions like anxiety, anger and sadness. Because these emotions were designed to be intense and uncomfortable, they often trigger a reflexive struggle to avoid or suppress them. We tighten up, grit our teeth, and breathe shallowly, if at all. Struggling with an emotion, however, tends to further inflame the emotion and related suffering. This struggle is typically automatic and going on behind the scenes. We are not standing there thinking, 'I am uncomfortable with this emotion so I am going to fight with it!' It is something that happens when we are on autopilot.

But we can learn to become aware of when we are experiencing emotional distress. We can tune in to the fact that we are suffering. Then, we can slow down — even for a few seconds (or pause for a moment) in order to buy the precious time we need to rein in our automatic (autopilot) reaction. Only then can we choose how we respond to the moment.

SKILL BUILDING: MINDFUL PAUSE

In this simple exercise you practise pausing and checking in with how you are doing. Learning to stop and check in with yourself is essential for the mindful awareness of distress, which is needed to help you slow down and get off autopilot. If you have ever come home after a long day and only then realized that you had been tense and stressed, this can be a very helpful practice. With the regular practice of pausing and checking in with yourself during the day you can develop this very helpful mindful habit.

- To begin, set up a regular reminder to get your attention once per hour during the day. If you are using your phone or smart watch, you can set it to vibrate hourly. If you would prefer not to use technology, you can build these mindful slowing and checking-in breaks into your day by tying them in with activities you routinely do such as driving, catching public transport, walking your dog, eating a meal, or using the bathroom. Perhaps you could leave a note on your refrigerator that says 'Time for a check-in.'
- When you are cued to check in, notice whether it is safe to take a brief time-out from your daily hectic pace (you're not a firefighter battling a blaze right now). Then slow down or pause your current activity. Take a couple of slow, deep breaths. Let go of any extra tension you are carrying around in your body.
- Notice what has been happening without your awareness. Notice if you are rushing or engaged in an activity with a

sense of urgency? Are you tensing muscles, gritting your teeth, or holding your breath? Are you doing something right now that runs counter to your value system?

- Next, see if you can briefly take helpful action. If you are walking or talking with pressured speed, go slow for a moment and notice what that feels like. If you are holding your breath, breathe slowly and deeply. If you are clenching your muscles tightly out of stress, invite those muscles to ease as much as they are willing. Then, return to the task at hand or shift to a more values-based activity. Depending on the situation, you can continue being slower and more mindful, if you'd like.

KEY POINTS

- Noticing you are suffering can be a signal that you may also be on autopilot.

- Practising mindful check-ins can help you learn to notice when you are experiencing suffering.

- Then slow down to buy yourself time (even seconds) to get centred and in control once again.

3

SETTING AN INTENTION TO DO WHAT IS HELPFUL

Something has happened. And now you are feeling painful emotions and have strong urges to react based on your threat instincts.

- 'I can't tolerate this social discomfort — I have to leave now!'
- 'He is disrespecting me — and I need to teach that guy a lesson!'
- 'I can't tolerate a panic attack. I must fight it or it will make me pass out!'

These powerful instincts are trying to take charge of you by producing a powerful urge to react impulsively. Acting on these urges, however, can lead to increased interpersonal and emotional turmoil. For example, yelling at your spouse when angry leads to a strained relationship, or avoiding a desired social event because of anxiety increases your fear of such events in the future and decreases your social opportunities.

You've taken a moment to slow down — but you're not quite off autopilot yet. You are still highly distressed. What do you do?

The problem is that it can be very difficult to think clearly when you suddenly find yourself highly distressed. And it doesn't help matters that your threat system is fighting with you over control of yourself. It is okay if you are not sure right here and now what to do. You are experiencing a moment of suffering and you can set an intention to try to do something helpful, even though you're not yet sure what to do.

Whatever you choose to do, it makes sense to do something that eases suffering and is consistent with how you would like to live your life. By setting a helpful intention you are beginning to open the door to taking action that addresses suffering in a way that's consistent with your values.

In the heat of the moment, however, you might catch yourself trying to set a helpful intention using a harsh critical tone: 'Do something helpful, dammit! Don't you screw this up!' Sadly, people too often talk to themselves in this way, even during better moments. The problem is that speaking to yourself in a threatening way further revs up your threat system. That's going in the wrong direction during a time that already feels highly threatening.

The better option is to begin to open the door to the soothing and centring power of compassion. We will do a deep dive into compassion a bit later, but for now you can see how setting a helpful intention from an inner tone that is more gentle, warm and caring can help disengage your autopilot that is itching to take over and drive your life.

Using a compassionate tone to fuel your helpful intent

Imagine someone you care deeply about. Now imagine they are experiencing an emotionally painful moment. Let's say, for example, they are terrified to fly, but have pushed themselves to take a flight with you. The plane hits heavy turbulence early into the flight and you notice that they are feeling incredibly distressed. You would likely have the intention to do something helpful for them, like letting them know how brave they are to face their fear.

Think about how you would speak to them while they are suffering on the flight. Rather than speaking to them in a neutral or hostile way, you would most likely use a warm and supportive tone. People naturally do this with the people they care most about because instinctively they know that a kind, warm tone can help buffer someone's distress.

Unfortunately, people can naturally default to a harsh or critical inner-tone when it comes to their own suffering — increasing their distress. With practice, however, you can learn to intentionally shift your inner tone to one of warmth and encouragement. That's not to say that a compassionate tone will fully eradicate a raging emotional storm. Rather, a compassionate tone can help you centre yourself and ease your sense of suffering while experiencing emotional distress. It can also activate the part of the nervous system designed to soothe distress (the parasympathetic nervous system).[1] This can help ground you while you turn to face the difficult moment.

Now, let's practise shifting into a compassionate tone.

SKILL BUILDING: COMPASSIONATE TONE

In this exercise we'll directly practise generating a compassionate inner tone.

Let's start with an experiment. Let's notice what it feels like to experience a hostile tone, a neutral tone, and a warm, kind tone. You can keep your eyes opened or closed for this.

- In your mind, say your name ten times. Use a tone as if you are talking to someone you are angry or disappointed with. Leave a space of a second or two between each time you say your name. Afterwards, review what you felt: What did your muscles do? Did your breathing change? People are often surprised by how painful this can be — yet during difficult moments they may default to a harsh tone in their self-talk just by reflex.
- For the second round, say your name ten times neutrally, as if you are reading the contents of your grocery list. Space them apart by a second or two. Did you notice a difference in how you felt?
- Now for the final round, think of an old friend, family member or favourite pet that you care deeply about. Imagine you have not seen them in a while as you have been away on a long trip. Say your name with the same warmth and kindness you would direct towards them when they meet you at the airport after your long trip. You can even allow yourself to have a gentle smile on your face as you do this. Again, space each repetition of your name apart by a second or two.

What did you notice? If you are like most, you may have been at least a bit surprised by how painful a harsh inner tone can feel relative to the warm and kind tone. It's quite a difference. A more compassionate tone can be your go-to strategy at the first sign of inner turmoil. This is similar to how you might approach a close friend who is dealing with something challenging: 'I'm sorry you're going through that, Sue. How can I help?'

I invite you to practise directing a compassionate tone towards yourself when you are struggling with a challenge or just because it is a pleasant and helpful thing to do. The more you practise this, the more ready you'll be to come to your own assistance with a more compassionate tone during those all-too-frequent times when life gets difficult.

SKILL BUILDING:
COMPASSIONATE TOUCH

> Compassion researcher, Dr Kristen Neff, advocates adding compassionate touch to help bolster ourselves during difficult moments.[2] Why is this helpful? We are designed from the very start of life until our last breath to be soothed by a caring touch. When a baby is crying in distress what does the empathic carer do in response? Go to the child, pick them up, and hold them gently. Even as we get older, what do we do for our loved ones who have just had a tremendous loss or disappointment? We hug them or put a caring hand gently on their shoulder (and speak to them in kind and gentle tones).

THE MINDFUL FREAK-OUT

Some people find adding compassionate self-touch, such as placing their hand on their heart or shoulder, can also help turn down the sting from painful emotions and help bring the strength and wisdom needed to override the threat system's powerful attempts at taking over.

Other people may find this uncomfortable for a number of reasons (See Chapter 14, 'Fears, blocks, and resistances to compassion') and if that is you, you are welcome to try compassionate touch or skip this altogether.

- If you are willing, try this right now and then you can practise it whenever you feel even a little distressed (or at any time just to practise being supportive). Take a moment and think of something in your life that is mildly challenging.
- Now place a hand gently and supportively on your chest over your heart — or a supportive hand on your own shoulder. Feel the warmth and support. As you do so, direct a kind, warm tone towards yourself. The attitude to strive for is, 'In this difficult moment I've got your back; I'm here for you right now'. Allow yourself to take in the sense of support and care that the touch communicates.

By this point in the book, you have learned to notice when you are experiencing a painful emotion, slow down your reaction, and bring a compassionate tone towards yourself as you set an intention to handle a painful moment in a helpful way.

In the next chapter we will focus on anchoring your attention to the present moment — further shutting off autopilot — so you can begin to face the moment in a more effective way.

KEY POINTS

- Once you realize you are suffering, set an intention to handle this situation in a helpful (not harmful) way.

- Using a compassionate inner tone and touch can help you begin to sooth your suffering and begin to shift your mindset from one of threat-reacting to one of helpful-responding.

4

ANCHORING YOUR ATTENTION IN THE PRESENT MOMENT

Another effective strategy for getting off autopilot when your threat emotions try to take control of you is to anchor your attention in the here and now. Painful emotions will try to pull your attention every which way. You might find yourself ruminating about something that happened in the past (for example, replaying an encounter with someone who was rude to you!) or your attention might get focused on the future, leading you to worry about what could happen *then*.

- 'What if I have a panic attack!'
- 'What if I get rejected!'
- 'What if I let him get away with that!'

Given that you have zero control over the past, and the future is always uncertain, a more helpful focus of attention is to come back to the present moment. This is the place where you can begin to work to ease your suffering. For example, let's say you had a bout of insomnia and spent last night tossing and turning. Your alarm clock goes off as you realize with great dread that it is time to go to work. Your anxiety grabs your attention and ruminates over how 'terrible' it was that you couldn't sleep. It reminds you over and over of what it was like to struggle in bed all night feeling uncomfortable, anxious and worried. Then your mind goes into fortune-telling mode, bringing your attention to catastrophic thoughts about the day ahead.

Most of this is happening automatically — you are on autopilot. In order to disengage your autopilot you will benefit from corralling your attention to the present moment.

We do this using 'mindfulness' which, according to writer and professor of medicine Dr Jon Kabat-Zinn, is the practice of intentionally paying attention to the present moment without judgment.[1] While your mind is a non-stop chatterbox, you are not the stories your mind creates for you. Yet those stories can be so distressing that they hijack your attention, body and behaviours. Mindfulness can help you to pull back from the story and see that you and your life are separate from the running commentary in your mind.

If you are distressed by the consequence of having had insomnia the prior night, you can learn to come back to the present moment and notice that (without the struggle) the sleep deprivation actually makes you feel relaxed along with being tired. You can notice that your cup of warm coffee drunk mindfully is soothing and delicious — certainly compared to what might usually be the mindless swallowing of coffee while rushing out the door. And on the drive to work, you can mindfully observe things you have not noticed in quite some time. The sunrise is awe inspiring. The car seat is the most comfortable seat you own. The music on the car radio is a masterful work of art. And the smell of the cherry blossoms outside your office is the second-best smell you know (the coffee being the first).

ACT encourages you to 'contact the present moment' in this way so that you can begin to pull back from over-identifying with the stories your minds tells you ('I didn't sleep; it will be a horrible day!'). Instead, you can notice your experiences as a curious observer rather than struggling with and getting hooked by your brain's mental noise. In other words, mindfulness helps us get out of our minds and into our lives.[2]

With today's frenetic pace of life, bringing your attention back to the present moment can be difficult. There are social media posts to keep up with, breaking news to follow, emails, texts and various messaging to monitor and respond to. And that's just a drop in the bucket of all the stimuli competing for your attention. On top of this, perceived (or misperceived) threats that are in the past ('I didn't sleep at all last night!') or anticipated for the future ('I won't be able to function at all!') are extremely powerful magnets for your attention. All of this can make anchoring your attention in the present moment a skill that takes some practice to develop.

Anchoring your attention on your breathing

Your breathing is a convenient focus for mindfulness practice. It is something you are doing all the time anyway. With mindfulness, you are simply paying attention to it. CFT teaches people mindful focusing on the breath in order to centre themselves in the present moment and to deepen and pace their breath as a way to help soothe suffering in the moment. This is called soothing rhythm breathing.[3] Soothing rhythm breathing is the opposite of the rapid, shallow, dysregulated breathing that often accompanies distressing moments and serves to further crank up your nervous system. The quick, shallow breathing is good when survival is on the line, but not so good when you are dealing with the barrage of modern stressors.

Slowing and deepening your breath has been shown to be of both physical and emotional benefit. It increases heart-rate variability (which is related to better health and less depression, anxiety and stress). It can help bring some calm when life gets difficult by activating the parasympathetic nervous system.[4]

Mindful breathing is a very helpful action to take when you are caught in an emotional tsunami. It is like having a readily available life jacket to help keep you above water in the storm. By using your breath as an anchor to the present moment, you can re-centre yourself during a difficult moment while beginning to bring soothing to meet your suffering.

In other words, breathe mindfully — suffer less. Breathe with mindless dysregulation — crank up your distress.

SKILL BUILDING: SOOTHING RHYTHM BREATHING

Here is a mindful soothing rhythm breathing exercise adapted from CFT:[5]
- Give yourself permission to let go of the day's mental noise

and find a comfortable seated position where you are fully supported. Allow muscle tension to soften as much as it is willing. If it is comfortable for you, you can allow your eyes to close — or alternatively, allow the gaze to focus on a neutral spot in front of you.
- Bring your attention to your breath just as it is. Notice it flowing in and watch it flow back out. You may notice that the air feels a bit cooler when you inhale and a bit warmer when you exhale. Inevitably, you will notice that your mind gets distracted and your attention is pulled away from breath and into various thoughts, images and memories. This is normal — that's what minds do. When you notice that your attention has left your breath, gently bring it back. If this happens repeatedly, it is okay — gently bring it back each time.
- Now, when you inhale, invite your breath down into your stomach, gently inflating your stomach. Then, when you breathe out, allow your stomach to settle back down. Bring your attention to rest on the rising and settling of your stomach as you breathe in and breathe out. Find a smoothness and steady rhythm in the flow of your breath.
- You might notice that as you pay attention to your breathing it begins to slow. See if you can invite that slowness to deepen. As you inhale, count out 3 seconds, then hold your breath for one second, and exhale for another count of three. After a few breaths see how it feels to increase your inhale to 4 seconds, hold for one, and release for 4 seconds. Give that a few breaths. Then inhale for 5 seconds,

THE MINDFUL FREAK-OUT

    hold for one, and release for 5 seconds.
- Once you have found a smooth and comfortable pace for your breath, give yourself a few minutes to practise. When your mind wanders, note it kindly and guide it back to the breath. Feel free to stay with this as long or as short as you would like. When you are ready, give yourself time to slowly open your eyes and return your focus to the sights, sounds and feel of your body in the room.

It seems that there are countless breathing strategies and most of the adults I work with have tried mindful breathing of some sort. Breathing exercises can be a bit like trying on shoes of different sizes to see what fits you well. What seems most important is that you find a pace that feels good to you.

Some like to keep it as barebones as possible. If this is you, instead of counting breaths you might prefer to just inhale deeply into the stomach and then focus your attention on extending your exhale, letting it linger longer than the inhale.

Some people feel uncomfortable when focusing on their breathing at all. If this is the case for you, it is okay to choose a different mindfulness anchoring practice. We will discuss several.

Please keep in mind that the goal of soothing rhythm breathing (and present moment awareness strategies, in general) is not to force your painful emotion into submission. Approaching with that agenda will likely backfire. It is about grounding yourself (and easing your suffering) in the present moment so that you regain control over yourself from the threat system — rather than the threat system controlling you.

SKILL BUILDING:
SENSORY AWARENESS TRAINING

For this exercise, you will learn to use your five senses as an effective way to become mindfully grounded in the present moment. This can serve you well when your threat system is howling.

- Take a couple of minutes to engage in soothing rhythm breathing.
- Now, look around for a minute and notice where you are. What do you see? Notice people and things in your environment. Notice the shapes and colours of the objects. If there is a window or if you are outside, notice the sights of nature: the grass, trees, the clouds and sky. Try to notice one thing in your environment that you've never really noticed before. Even if you are in your childhood home where you were raised, you can notice something you have never noticed before — perhaps a cobweb on the ceiling, details in a picture hanging on the wall, or the pattern on the leaves of a houseplant.
- Next, pay attention to what you can feel with your body. Notice your feet on the ground and the texture beneath them. Notice the weight of your body on the furniture you are sitting or reclining on. Notice the texture of the material on that surface. Notice how hard or soft it is. Notice the feeling of the clothes on your body — are they tight or loose? Feel the air temperature and any air movement around you.
- Notice the sounds in your environment. What are the

sounds you can hear that are nearby? What sounds can you hear that are further away? How many different sounds can you identify? Is there a sound you can now notice that you were not aware of before? Are there subtle variations in the sounds you can detect?
- If you have a drink or a snack near you, bring it close and notice the aroma. What can you observe? Taste a small amount. Savour the subtle flavours.

A quick and easy variation to the above sensory awareness exercise is to use the '5, 4, 3, 2, 1 method':

Notice and name 5 things you can see.

Notice and name 4 things you can feel with your body.

Notice and name 3 things you can hear.

Notice and name 2 things you can smell.

Notice and name 1 thing you can taste.

Notice what it is like to be fully present in your life right here and now — when and where it is actually happening. When your mind drags you into the past or future, respond by gently redirecting your attention back to the present moment. It is not helpful to try to push away your uncomfortable emotions or thoughts of the past or future (which can make them paradoxically more sticky and prickly). Rather, you are using your senses to turn off autopilot and orient yourself to what is helpful for you right now.

SKILL BUILDING:
USING YOUR BODY FOR MINDFUL AWARENESS

> It can also help you to come back to the present moment if you move your body for a moment. For example, you can take a long slow stretch, as if you've just woken up. Or try gently but firmly pressing your feet onto the floor. Maybe even shake off the autopilot by shaking your arms. These strategies are not meant to be used as a distraction or other emotionally avoidant tactic. They are intended to wake you up to what you are experiencing and begin to ground yourself in the moment.
>
> If you practise yoga, picking an easily accessible pose or two to move through in conjunction with your breath is an excellent use of your body, to help anchor yourself in the present moment. If available to you, you can increase your sensory awareness using safe yet strong physical sensations such as drinking a frosty cold or comfortably warm beverage, or holding an ice cube and mindfully watching and feeling it melt. If time and context permit, you could briskly exercise or perhaps take a warm or chilly shower using a water temperature that focuses your attention in the present moment.

Have you ever had a day when you didn't realize how stressed you were until the day was almost over? Perhaps after work you noticed a tension headache or an upset stomach that you had been too busy or distracted to notice at the time. Did you ever suddenly realize you had been holding your breath or breathing very shallowly from anger or anxiety? We are often so distracted by modern life that we lose touch with what is happening physically and emotionally throughout the day. It happens all the time.

This lack of awareness can be problematic if you miss the early signs that you are building towards a tipping point. Have you ever snapped at a loved one only then to realize, 'Oh, I am feeling irritable today'? Perhaps you turned down a social invitation then later realized, 'I was feeling anxious'. People can be unaware of their building emotions, growing in the background, only to become aware once a full-blown panic attack or angry outburst has developed.

Likewise, people may not realize they are locked into a hidden war with their emotions, attempting to defeat those emotions with food, knock them out with a mind-altering substance, or distract from them by mindlessly scrolling through social media. Many walk around unconsciously trying to crush their emotions with brute force by squeezing their muscles uncomfortably tight (only later to suffer from muscle pain or other tension-induced problems). Those behaviours are often driven by autopilot.

SKILL BUILDING:
MINDFUL AWARENESS OF EMOTIONS

Beginning to wake up to the reality of what you are feeling, without judgment, can buy you the precious time and space needed to respond in a wise way. For that, practising mindful awareness of emotions can help.

Let's practise:

- Take a moment to slow down and pause your day for a moment. Allow yourself to get in touch with your breathing and find that soothing rhythm that's slower, deeper and more comfortable for you (see p. 42 for a refresher). Breathe down into your stomach if that feels okay for you. Give yourself a minute or two to do this. As always, you can feel free to close your eyes or allow them to remain open and focused on something neutral, like the wall or the floor.
- Now, recall a time you spent with friends or loved ones that was enjoyable. Imagine you get to relive this.
  - What do you see?
  - Who is present with you?
  - Notice their facial expressions and how they are behaving towards you.
  - Notice the sounds of their voices and, if you are outside, the sounds of nature around you.
- Notice and name the dominant emotion you feel right now.
  - Focus inwardly and see where in your body you notice this feeling.
  - What sensations do you feel physically in your body pertaining to that emotion?
  - How much space does it take up in your body?
  - Are there shapes or colours associated with the sensations?
  - Do the emotions have a certain texture to them?
  - Do they stay the same as you focus on them or do they change in any way?

THE MINDFUL FREAK-OUT

- See if you can hold the emotion softly in your body.
  - When your mind wanders, that's normal; gently redirect your mind back to how you experience the emotion in your body.
  - Notice if the emotion leads to any urges or desires. If so, name them.
- Now, notice any thoughts that come to mind. Watch them come and go in their own time.
- Return to focusing on your breathing for a moment. Slowly and smoothly breathe in and out. Give yourself a minute of breathing focus.
- Now, let's do something more challenging. Think of a time you felt an uncomfortable emotion, like anxiety, sadness or irritability. If you are just starting out, pick something that is only mildly triggering.
  - Recall the incident in your imagination: see what you saw and hear what you heard.
  - Now, focus on where you feel the associated emotion in your body.
  - Notice the shape and size of the emotion.
  - Where does it start and where does it end?
  - Notice if there are specific colours or textures associated with the emotion.
  - See if it remains stable, or does it change as you focus on it?
  - Notice whether you are opening softly to make space for the emotion or whether you are bracing against the emotion. Has the emotion changed your quality of breathing?

- Notice if your mind is wandering or whether you are distracting yourself by focusing on something more pleasant. Either of those are natural and understandable – and see if you can gently direct your attention back to the emotion in your body.
- Breathe the emotion in and breathe out the struggle against the emotion. See if you can bring some gentle curiosity to your experience of the emotion.
- After a few minutes, set the imagery aside, take a few more rhythmic breaths, allow your eyes to open if they were closed, and come back to the room you are in.

By doing this exercise, I hope you had the experience of being able to sit with and observe your emotions without becoming overwhelmed or taken over by them. Did you notice that resisting the emotion can happen automatically and when you catch and release the struggle, the emotion typically feels less distressing?

An alternative emotional mindfulness exercise is to follow the same instructions, but instead of using past memories to stimulate the emotion you can watch a short video on the internet that brings out the emotions. For anger, pick your least favourite politician and play a video of them at a rally. For sadness, you can pick a scene from a tearjerker film. And for anxiety, you can play a scene from a horror movie, or a video filled with creepy spiders, or perhaps just peruse the latest news stories.

Turning on your observing mind

Have you ever noticed that throughout your life there is always a part of you that just sits back and notices what's happening? All day our brains are telling us stories ('content' such as 'I'm too anxious to go to the dinner party'). Some of these stories are helpful, especially those that motivate action that is important to you (e.g. 'If you don't study for your test, you won't pass it'). Other stories, not so much ('You're unlovable … why even try a dating app?').

Often, people are attached to the various stories their mind tells them and behave as if the stories are true and important, even when they are not. Part of getting off autopilot is realizing that your threat system creates stories which are not helpful. For example, another driver cuts you off in traffic and your mind activates the story about you needing 'to teach them a lesson!' and if the story hooks you, then you speed up, honk your horn and hurl insults directed at their mother — and all of this taking place on your drive to church because you value peace and compassion.

There is a part of you, however, that transcends the stories your mind generates. ACT calls this the 'self-as-context' or the observing mind. It is the part of you that notices life as it is happening, even in the heat of the moment. There is the part of you that notices:

'Wow, I'm really feeling angry and out of control right now.'
'I'm anxious and uncomfortable.'
'I'm just lying around feeling sad.'
'I am having so much fun hanging out with my friends.'

The observing self has always been with you — it is stable. The *you* that noticed that you felt sad because your mother left the room when you were a toddler is the same *you* that noticed feeling sad when your friend didn't respond to your text.

People often get caught up in their stories. They can confuse who they are with the stories their minds can tell them. Take the thought, 'I'm an anxious person'. Do you cease to be you when you feel peaceful or angry? It can help you get off autopilot when you get in touch with that stable part of you who sits back in your mind and observes 'I am really anxious'. You can observe this mental story with gentle curiosity: 'Huh, I am aware that my anxiety is rising and my brain is telling me stories'. If you can step back and get off autopilot, you have a choice in how you want to respond. If you are fused with the content, you are more likely to be swept away by these stories.

By practising dropping into your observing mind, it will be easier to access when emotional distress is high. By practising this, you can learn to step back into this perspective, in the heat of a highly distressing moment, which can help buy you the very precious space to choose your response in the difficult moment.

SKILL BUILDING: BEING THE NOTICER

> You can do this exercise anywhere and anytime. Just notice something and notice who is noticing. I'm typing on my computer right now and I can notice myself noticing my typing. I notice the sky is light blue – and I notice my noticing. I notice an orchestra of birds tweeting throughout the neighbourhood – and I notice I'm noticing. I notice my back

feels sore against the hard wooden chair — and I notice the urge to move — and I notice my noticing. I notice a faint floral aroma in the air — and I am aware of my noticing. I am also aware of the aftertaste of dark chocolate in my mouth — and I notice my noticing.

The point is to mindfully engage your senses, as you have practised above, but now you are taking one step further back to illuminate the stable inner noticer that has been part of you your entire life.

Can you notice yourself noticing that you are reading the words on this page? When you go for that snack later can you step into that part of you that observes your experience of craving and then eating the snack? Or perhaps you could take a mindful walk while noticing yourself noticing the walk. As you practise this skill, see if you can start to notice the autopilot more often. Once you notice it, you increase your ability to disengage it.

Formal mindfulness-based exercises are well researched and in addition to helping you get better at getting off autopilot they offer numerous other physical and mental health benefits.[6] However, some people may already feel overloaded with demands on their time. Life can get hectic.

The good news is that mindfulness can be practised without any additional time requirements. Zero. The formula for this is to simply *notice what you are doing when you are doing it*. Take something you do daily like brushing your teeth. You can choose to fiddle with your phone with one hand while brushing with the other, while having a semi-coherent conversation with your partner or child (no, you are not the only one who does this).

Or you can choose to practise focusing on brushing your teeth while you are brushing your teeth.

SKILL BUILDING:
INCORPORATING PRESENT MOMENT AWARENESS INTO YOUR DAILY ROUTINE

> Notice what you see: the shape and colour of the brush, the colour and writing on the toothpaste tube, the sight of the toothpaste spreading onto the bristles of your brush, and the sight of the brush as it moves towards your open mouth.
>
> Notice what you hear: background sounds in the environment, the sound of the brush whisking back and forth around your teeth, the sound of the water dripping from the tap, the sound of the water sloshing around your mouth, and then the sound of the water when you spit into the sink.
>
> Notice what you feel: the weight of the tube of toothpaste in your hand, the feel of the ridged cap in your fingers, the feel of the tube of paste in one hand being squeezed while noticing the slight weight of the toothbrush in your other hand. Notice the gentle massage of the brush bristles on your teeth, like a mini massage. Then feel the influx of water as it moves into, around and then back out of your mouth. Notice what it feels like to breathe slowly and

THE MINDFUL FREAK-OUT

>   gently while you are brushing your teeth.
> - Notice what you smell and taste: the aroma of the toothpaste and the flavour within your mouth.
> - As you brush your teeth mindfully, your mind will be pulled this way and that. You'll have the urge to read your emails, listen to music, or daydream about anything more interesting than brushing your teeth. When you notice that your mind is no longer thinking about brushing your teeth, congratulate yourself — you just came back into awareness and can gently redirect your attention back to the tooth brushing. It is important to not judge yourself harshly when your mind wanders — it is designed to do so and is not your fault! Kindly shepherd your attention back to the task at hand over and over.

And there you go. You just did a mindful awareness training exercise that, over time, can add to your physical and mental health, with zero added time to your day. You can expand this practice to other activities like driving your car to the supermarket without turning on music or talking on the phone. Just focus on the sensory experience of driving in the moment.

Which other daily activities could you practise with? Perhaps mundane chores like washing the dishes or folding laundry. Perhaps you could use it to savour activities like mindful awareness of eating or drinking a favourite food or beverage. You can practise being more present when you are playing with your kids or chatting with a loved one or giving (or receiving) a backrub. You can tune into the sensory experience of nature when you go for your weekly hike. Do as much or as little as works for you. You can start with one very small practice and build up if you'd like.

Going from compassionate awareness to compassionate acceptance

Learning to sit back and observe what is happening around you and inside you can help you wake up to the challenges of the present moment, enabling you to disengage your autopilot and take back control of your own actions. In Part 2, you will learn to ease your suffering by facing your experience with compassion, letting go of struggle, and unhooking from unhelpful thoughts. This can be invaluable in helping you respond to painful emotions in a way that is consistent with your values rather than gut emotional reactions.

KEY POINTS

- Your threat system can pull your attention away from the present moment, how you are feeling, and what is important to you.

- Mindfulness can help you centre in the present moment, freeing you up to choose how you wish to respond to a difficult moment.

- There are many ways to practise mindfulness: you can focus on your senses, emotions, physical sensations, and your breathing.

THE MINDFUL FREAK-OUT

- Slow, deep, mindful breathing can also help you calm down and re-centre.

- Practising noticing your observing mind can also help you centre and anchor in the present moment.

PART 2

FACING PAINFUL MOMENTS WITH COMPASSION

(Compassionate Acceptance)

5

THE PROBLEM WITH FIGHTING YOUR FEELINGS

Many of us spend much of our lives trying not to feel the variety of painful emotions that life presents. We distract, we struggle, we fight. Anything not to feel emotional pain. Yet here we are — still distracting, still struggling, and still fighting emotions that bounce back even stronger. It is like the mythological Hydra, the multi-headed beast. You cut off a head and two more grow back in its place. We keep searching for a way to be forever free of painful moments only to be disappointed again and again. Frustrating, isn't it?

The case for acceptance

Increasing your acceptance of something as painful as intense, unpleasant emotions seems like a lot to ask. However, I hope you will give me the opportunity of your attention a bit longer so I can show you why 'acceptance' might not be what you think it is.

Your instinct to run from or fight painful emotions makes sense. Who wouldn't want to avoid feeling emotionally uncomfortable? However, struggling to avoid painful emotions comes with a number of risks.

1. You'll inevitably fail. Human life is chock full of all kinds of intense emotions — many of them painful.
2. The best things in life involve emotional pain at some points (love, for example, means being vulnerable to being hurt; no hurt = no love).
3. Struggling to get rid of painful thoughts and feelings tends to throw fuel on the emotional fire — further igniting their intensity.

Let's experiment: observing the consequence of emotional struggle

When it comes to painful emotions, people often struggle with the thoughts and physical sensations that make up painful emotions. Let's see what happens when you try this.

Struggling with distressing thoughts

Think of something that is at least a little distressing. It doesn't need to be something that provokes high anxiety, but something that wakes up an uncomfortable emotion. See if you can come up with a word or a phrase that captures the essence of your concern. If you are anxious regarding an upcoming test, you could use 'test' or 'final exam', for example.

Set a timer for 60 seconds. Try for a minute to eradicate the uncomfortable thought from your mind. Your objective is to get rid of the anxious thought. Imagine your life depended upon it. Get ready. Go!

Make sure the thought is gone. Don't think of anything even remotely related to it. Is it gone? Are you absolutely sure? Keep it up for the entire minute. Don't think about _____. Don't think about it. If it shows up, even for a moment, fight with all you have to forever vanquish the thought!

Time's up. What did you notice? If you are like most, you noticed that the harder you fought the thoughts the louder and stickier those thoughts became. Struggle intensified them.

Now let's try the opposite. Set your timer for 60 seconds. This time invite the thought to be there, with your permission. Allow it to be background noise while letting go of any struggle. Just breathe and allow. Neither attend to it nor push it away. Just let it be there for the minute.

How was that different? If you are like most, you may have realized that without actively wrestling with the thought, it became somewhat less interesting and perhaps even faded from your mind. Which of the two, struggle versus acceptance, led to less suffering?

Struggling with uncomfortable feelings
Now let's try another experiment. Once again bring to mind the mildly distressing situation. Allow the uncomfortable emotion to increase by thinking about the situation for a moment.

I invite you to take 60 seconds and tighten your body as if you were trying to squeeze the emotion out of your body (this is what we often do as we tense up in reaction to distress). Tightly squeeze your muscles, being careful not to exacerbate any medical conditions you might have.

Tighten your jaw, furrow your brow, squeeze your stomach. Make fists and hold them in front of you tightly. At the same time, squeeze your legs and feet.

As you tighten, notice how you are no longer breathing smoothly. Notice how the fight impacts your level of suffering. What do you feel emotionally? Does it make you feel frustrated or annoyed? Does it lower your distress or raise it?

It is like those finger traps we played with as children. Put a finger into each end of the woven tube, then the harder you try to tug your fingers apart, the tighter the tube squeezes — making you more stuck!

Now let's try the opposite. Bring to mind the distressing situation. Then, open your fists and gently lay the back of your open hands on your lap or along your sides. Let go of muscle tension throughout the body. Let go of struggling in your feet, legs, stomach, arms, chest, back, neck, jaw and around your eyes. Just let yourself feel what is there, willingly and gently. How is that different? If you are like most, you'll have found that letting go allowed for greater soothing and centring, even in the face of the unpleasant emotion.

The bottom line is that acceptance brings less suffering than struggle.

The ACT of acceptance

ACT uses 'acceptance' as a springboard to a better life. It recognizes that anything or anyone you care about might lead to painful emotions at times:

- **Your teen is two hours late and is not answering their phone.**

- You are being interviewed for your dream job. You really want this job, but recognize you might not get it if the interview doesn't go well.
- Going to university means lots of anxiety-provoking exams.
- The person on the dating app you were excited about asked you out. Meeting in person means things could go wrong — they might not like you and meeting for the first time will feel awkward.

Acceptance does not mean that you *want* to feel uncomfortable — few of us like discomfort. Acceptance is an alternative to avoiding or struggling with your experience. It involves being aware of and embracing what your thoughts and feelings bring to you in a given moment, rather than treating them like an enemy and increasing your suffering. And, it is about pursuing a life that is important to you, even though it is sometimes painful.

The Devil's bargain

I heard Steven Hayes talk about 'The Devil's bargain' during a lecture, and I am loosely paraphrasing his anecdote.

The Devil approaches you during a day filled with anxiety and stress. He flashes you a slick smile and says, 'How'd you like me to remove all the stress and anxiety from your life?' He assures you, 'I can make it so that your life stays comfortable. What do you say?'

You think about your stressful day and how nice it would feel to never worry about things. However, as this is the Devil, you suspect there is a catch. You ask and he grins, 'Well, for starters, you'll have to give up everything and everyone you care about. You can't strive for an education or career, you can't have friends, you can't have family or really any attachments at all. You'll have to give up any future ambition. If you don't give a damn about anything then you don't have anything of value to worry or feel bad about.

'And you'll lose the ability to understand and empathize with the pain other humans experience. You'll be like an uncaring robot with zero desire, human connection or ambition of any kind. But you'll be stress-free. What'd you say? Are you ready to sign up for this?'

You can certainly choose the route of least discomfort in life by avoiding pursuing what matters most to you: the people and situations that feel important. However, if you choose to live a life based on what matters to you, learning to accept the painful thoughts and feelings that naturally show up can lead to a life you value, with less suffering.

The workability of avoiding emotional distress

From an ACT standpoint, trying to avoid or get rid of your painful thoughts and feelings versus accepting them is all about 'workability'. This means doing what moves you towards a rich, meaningful life. If acceptance allows you to move towards what is important to you (even in the face of emotional discomfort) that's a wonderful thing. If acceptance eases your suffering — so much better! ACT is all about living your life not based on avoidance of certain thoughts or feelings, but an active embrace of what shows up along the path towards a rich and values-based life. For example:

- **asking someone on a date while accepting the presence of fear of rejection**
- **going to university while accepting being anxious before exams**
- **having children while accepting the added financial stress.**

Acceptance absolutely *does not* mean accepting things that are changeable, things that will lead to a better life. If you are in an abusive relationship, an unrewarding job, or are lacking in skills needed to parent a challenging teen, you are encouraged to make changes that move you towards a better life (while accepting that those changes might come with initial distress). If caffeine makes you feel so jumpy that it is hard to focus on work, then feel free to ease up. However, if you are feeling jumpy because you have a date tonight, acceptance will lead to less suffering while you move towards your valued goal of finding love.

If you are being persecuted in the world, you can choose to fight like hell to change that situation. However, when the presence of your thoughts and emotions is what is persecuting you then acceptance, at least in the moment, will likely serve you better than fighting them.

THE MINDFUL FREAK-OUT

KEY POINTS

- We often hurt in life — especially around things we care deeply about.

- It is natural to want to struggle against painful thoughts and feelings; however, this makes them louder and increases suffering.

6

ENGAGING YOUR COMPASSIONATE MIND

Harnessing the power of compassion during life's most distressing moments

Compassion Focused Therapy is an evidence-based therapeutic approach to cultivating compassion and applying it to the problem of human suffering. It was created by Dr Paul Gilbert, a psychologist and researcher in the United Kingdom. He was originally trained in Cognitive Behavioural Therapy. Then one day he was helping one of his patients challenge her unhelpful thinking about a situation by using logic and reason. However, she pointed out that although she could logically understand the new thought, she didn't feel any better. He asked her about the tone she was using as she was talking to herself in her mind. She was being brutal towards herself in her own mind, harshly berating herself for being a bad therapy patient.

THE MINDFUL FREAK-OUT

Gilbert observed that even though she was technically correct in how she was using a therapeutic technique, the harsh tone in her mind kept her suffering cranked up high. That was his lightbulb moment. Human life is difficult at times and, unfortunately, we often treat ourselves (and sometimes others) in harsh or judgmental ways that compound suffering rather than work to ease it.

Think about how you talk to yourself when you make a mistake. Would you speak that way to someone you care deeply about?

In our darkest and most painful moments, we can behave towards ourselves in ways we would never dream of treating even our worst enemy. When you are freaking out, you are likely suffering. In those moments (if you have gotten off autopilot) you can choose to shift from a harsh, critical tone that exacerbates suffering to a more compassionate tone that is a soothing balm to your suffering.

Zuri is being introduced and will soon walk up to the podium to give her presentation in front of the packed room. She feels panicked! Public speaking has long terrified her. She has managed to avoid it throughout the early part of her career, but with her recent promotion, giving presentations is now unavoidable.

On the outside, she seems composed, but inside is another matter: 'Who the heck do you think you are? You are not smart enough, clever enough or attractive enough to teach anyone anything! What a joke! You are a total imposter! You're never going to get through this. Everyone will see you for the incompetent person you are!'

The result of this self-on-self verbal abuse is that she is now feeling even more anxious — and filled with shame. Her suffering has intensified as she slowly makes the walk to the podium.

Zuri's anxiety was bound to show up given her phobia of public speaking and her long history of avoidance. Rather than working to ease her suffering, her hostile tone has inflamed it many times over. Meeting her anxiety with compassion, instead of criticism, could have given her a boost of inner strength and encouragement while easing her suffering in the face of a highly distressing moment.

Benefits of cultivating compassion

CFT aims to build compassion for ourselves as well as others. Compassion directs us to take effective action to prevent or alleviate suffering. Often, it involves generating feelings of warmth, inner strength, courage and kindness — this is the good stuff that can help us feel safer and balance out our noisy threat system. At other times, however, it could mean generating feelings of anger in order to defend ourselves or others from an injustice.

Compassion is far from a new concept. Buddhists have been huge advocates for more than 2000 years. Actually, the cultivation of compassion is one of those key concepts that all the main religions of the world can agree is a good goal to strive for.

In more recent years, compassion has become a hot topic for scientists to research. It has been shown, by a growing body of research, to be associated with numerous psychological, physical and social benefits, including (but not limited to) an increase in:

- **feelings of wellbeing**
- **mindfulness**
- **the perception of social connectedness**
- **life satisfaction**
- **parasympathetic nervous system activity (soothing the nervous system)**
- **empathy**
- **creativity**
- **prosocial behaviour**
- **feelings of safeness and contentment.**

Research has also shown that compassion also decreases:
- **feelings of shame**
- **the sense of suffering**
- **depressive symptoms**
- **anxiety**
- **psychological distress**
- **self-criticism**
- **implicit racism**
- **interpersonal conflict**
- **stress reactivity.**[1]

Just imagine if the pharmaceutical companies could bottle that up!

With the CFT exercises in the next chapter you can begin to build up your compassionate mind. In this chapter, however, we'll explore some of the concepts that CFT teaches in order to set the stage for learning to be more compassionate.

Where does compassion come from?

Mother Nature wants life to survive on planet Earth. She uses, however, very different strategies to promote species survival. The sea turtle, for example, will lay a couple of thousand eggs in its life. Rather than scrimping and saving for turtle university, the sea turtle lays her eggs and abandons each and every one of her offspring. Maybe one or two will survive to adulthood. It is a dangerous world out there and laying massive quantities of eggs is how the sea turtle species persists.

Humans have an entirely different survival strategy. We have very few offspring and care deeply for them. Humans are born 'half-baked' so that our big-brained heads can fit through the narrow birth canal. That makes us helpless at the beginning of our lives. A newborn horse shortly after birth is prancing around the field with some innate skill, but newborn human babies are born little lumps of pooping, drooling vulnerability that are so uncoordinated they get startled when their own hands pass in front of their eyes.

Humans have a powerful instinct to care deeply for their offspring. We are coded for compassion. In fact, most human parents would readily protect their offspring with their own lives! Without compassion, those little awkward lumps — and the entirety of the human species — would not survive long.

Then, along the journey of life, we will continue to depend upon the compassion of others, teachers, friends and co-workers, postal carriers and firefighters to name just a few. And in the end, we will count on compassionate nurses and doctors to ease our suffering as we leave our earthly existence.

This compassionate instinct has been with us for all of human history. For most of the time that we humans have been on Earth, we were nomadic hunter-gatherers living in small tribes. We needed each other to survive the harsh prehistoric lives we led. If I had a successful hunt and found myself with a large amount of valuable protein and fat, it would have been beneficial for the survival of the tribe for me to share. Likewise, when I didn't have a successful hunt, but Grogg in the next cave did, it would be beneficial for the survival of the tribe for him to share. Without the tribe, we couldn't possibly have survived for long in the harsh and violent conditions of prehistoric life. Compassion for others was (and remains) vital for our survival and wellbeing. When we are deprived of human compassion, such as in the case of abuse or neglect, a wide range of physical and psychological consequences can occur, such as poorer mental health, physical health and quality of life.[2]

But what exactly is compassion?

CFT uses a Buddhist-informed definition of compassion: compassion is the sensitivity to suffering in oneself and others along with a commitment to try to alleviate and prevent it.

This points to two different sets of attributes or skills that are needed to be compassionate:

1. *Engaging* with suffering (turning towards suffering).
2. *Alleviating and preventing* suffering (taking helpful action).

Some people mistakenly think that compassion is a feeling, like love. That's wrong. Compassion is a motive that can come from a range of emotions. If you see a child has fallen into a river and is about to be swept away, the compassionate motive to jump in and rescue the child will likely be accompanied with panic and urgency. If you see someone you love being attacked, it is likely that anger will fuel your compassionate reaction. And if you are consoling a friend who has been diagnosed with a terminal illness, your compassionate motive is likely accompanied by great sadness. The emotion that comes with a compassionate motive is dependent upon the situation.

Engaging with suffering

To address suffering, first you need to turn towards it.

What does it take to turn towards your own or another's suffering rather than ignore it? CFT identifies six core attributes that help people turn towards suffering:[3]

1. SENSITIVITY TO SUFFERING: Sensitivity is being aware and open to the experience of suffering in yourself or another. We cannot turn towards suffering in a helpful way if we are not aware that we or someone else is suffering. Often, when people are highly distressed they are on autopilot, reacting on instinct with less awareness that they are experiencing a moment of suffering. In fact, people often rush around unaware that they or those around them are feeling stressed out.
2. SYMPATHY: In CFT, sympathy means being moved by our own or another's suffering. People can be aware of their own or another's suffering without being moved; for example, callously yelling at an unhoused person

with mental illness to 'Get a job!' Having sympathy means being emotionally open to our or another's pain.
3. MOTIVATION TO CARE FOR WELLBEING: It's not enough to be aware that you or another is suffering or to just be moved by that suffering. To be compassionate there must be motivation to do something to alleviate it or prevent it rather than turning away from it.
4. DISTRESS TOLERANCE: If compassion is going to involve facing painful emotions, then distress tolerance is needed. Imagine that a close friend's spouse has received the diagnosis of a terminal illness. To be there for your friend in a compassionate way, you would need to be able to tolerate the distress that your friend is experiencing as well as your own distress. Likewise, when you are experiencing your own highly distressing moment, it is necessary to be able to tolerate the initial intensity of the distress so that you can begin to use tools and strategies outlined in this book to reduce your suffering.

   Part of distress tolerance is understanding that highly distressing moments are just that, moments — and they will pass. We can learn to ground ourselves, even within painful waves of emotion. We can't often stop the waves, but we can learn to surf.
5. NON-JUDGMENT: Non-judgment refers to being able to understand how the complexity of human life leads people to feel a certain way or their lives to have turned out in a particular way — rather than simply sinking

into condemnation. For example, when you think of the unhoused person on the street abusing alcohol you might hook onto thoughts such as 'They should just get a job, the lousy, lazy …'. Instead, you could pull back for a broader view that understands they did not pick so many of the factors that led them to such a state. Perhaps they had a horrific, abusive childhood or have experienced mental illness. Non-judgment means understanding that people usually do the best they can with whatever life has randomly tossed their way. Some win the parental or genetic lottery and, sadly, many lose those lotteries in terribly unfair and unfortunate ways.

6. EMPATHY: Empathy is the ability to understand why we or someone else thinks, feels or behaves in specific ways. Imagine someone who texts 'How was your drive?' to their romantic partner who had a long drive to an out-of-town business meeting. When they don't hear back in an hour, they might begin to panic, their brain filled with catastrophic thoughts. If you knew their best friend was killed in a car accident a few years back, you could empathically understand just how distressing this situation would be. Empathy involves putting yourself in someone else's shoes to imagine life from their perspective. For ourselves, it means taking a step back and realizing that how we are thinking, feeling or behaving makes sense given our unique history. This is a big step towards letting go of negative judgment.

THE MINDFUL FREAK-OUT

Using specific skills for alleviating and preventing suffering

To address suffering it is not enough just to turn towards it. If you see someone drowning, are moved by their distress to where you dive into the ocean to save them, but you can't swim — that is not effective compassionate action. CFT recommends a number of skills that are aimed at harnessing the power of compassion for alleviating or preventing suffering.

Attention

This involves the ability to focus your attention on what is helpful.

When you feel under threat, be it from an approaching grizzly bear or small talk at a party, your attention naturally narrows to focus on the threat while blocking your attention from whatever else may also be going on. This is adaptive in the case of the rapidly approaching bear. That bear is an actual threat and getting distracted by the pretty flowers on the nearby bush could be a deadly mistake while you are being chased by the bear. However, focusing your attention on misperceived threats is problematic. If you are nervous on a first date, you might find your attention drawn to an internal focus ('How does my hair look, did I just say something stupid, what if they don't like me?'). Not only does this internal focus escalate anxious suffering, but you are missing out on what you want to focus on — your date. Mindfulness training exercises, like you practised earlier in the book, can help you get better at noticing when your attention has wandered to something unhelpful. Over time, mindfulness can build your proficiency at shifting your attention (like redirecting a spotlight) to what *you* want to be focusing on.

Imagery

You can harness the power of imagery to cultivate a more helpful mindset when you are suffering. When you simply imagine something, parts of your brain respond as if that thing were here in reality. See for yourself.

Take a moment and think of one of your absolute favourite foods. Just imagine that the delivery driver just dropped off this food for you. Imagine taking the warm box out of the bag and notice the aroma as you inhale the delicious smell. You open the box and you see that the food was perfectly prepared and is ready to be eaten. You bring the box to your nose for one more tasty whiff. Now imagine taking your utensil and bringing some of the food up to your mouth. Imagine what that first bite feels like in your mouth and how it tastes.

What do you notice about your mouth right now? If you are like me (who was imagining the perfect slice of hot, cheesy pizza) your mouth produced saliva to help you digest your delicious meal — which, sadly, is not real.

Likewise, if you take a moment and bring to mind someone you have had a conflict with, someone who you would least like to run into at a social event, your body then reacts in a vastly different way. Just imagining this activates feelings of dread or threat.

Your body reacts to what your brain imagines. Knowing this, you can learn to direct your imagination in ways that can tell your mind and body that you are okay right now — you are safe. When life brings you highly distressing moments (as life will), once you have disengaged your autopilot you can take a moment and engage your compassionate mind using imagery. This compassionate imagery can turn up your safeness dial while turning down your threat dial.

THE MINDFUL FREAK-OUT

Compassionate reasoning

Rather than emotionally reactive reasoning, this involves reasoning based on a compassionate mindset.

When you are presented with an emotionally challenging moment reasoning tends to be shaped by your current mental state. If the predominant emotion is sadness, your reasoning will be filtered through negativity and loss. If it is anxiety, your reasoning will be heavily influenced by danger. And if it is anger, your reasoning will be pulled towards themes of injustice and retribution. Early in my training at a veterans' hospital, I met 'John', who demonstrated this default response in his reaction to a road-rage incident.

> *John is a long-retired, combat-hardened Marine. He is enjoying his retirement and spending time with his wife of 40 years and babysitting his tiny granddaughter. He's driving to the supermarket to stock up on nappies for his granddaughter's upcoming visit when a guy zips in front of him, nearly hitting his car, and speeds ahead. John feels rage, which shapes his reasoning. He tells himself, 'I have to teach that son of a bitch a lesson! Who does that guy think he is that he can treat me this way? I'll show him! He'll regret ever having done that to me!' John proceeds to speed up, run the other driver off the road, take out a tyre iron and smash the man's window. Then he proceeds to beat the man nearly to death.*

Compassionate reasoning can be engaged by slowing down and taking a step back from the powerful, impulsive reasoning that comes to you when you are feeling highly distressed. It means taking a moment to centre yourself during the emotional storm so that you can face the moment with a more balanced mindset that is wiser and has the intent to make the situation better, rather than to inflame. When you engage your compassionate mind using the strategies in the next chapter, you will find that you can reason in a way that is more values-consistent rather than emotion-driven.

Compassionate behaviour

Rather than reacting impulsively based on your threat instincts, compassionate behaviour involves taking action designed to alleviate or prevent suffering.

Some people mistakenly think that compassionate behaviour is doing what is most comfortable. This isn't the case. If you have agoraphobia, for example, it is not compassionate behaviour to stay home where things are comfortable and familiar. That keeps you stuck and suffering. If you struggle with social anxiety, it is not compassionate to load up on alcohol before going to the party in order to be more comfortable — that doesn't allow you to learn that these social situations are safe. These are 'quick fixes' that ease discomfort in the moment, but prolong your suffering over time. And you may also miss out on living life based on what is truly important to you (friendships, romance and career, for example). In fact, compassionate behaviour often involves turning towards what's difficult and painful, in the short term. For example, getting sober, facing a fear, ending an abusive relationship or dealing with longstanding trauma.

Compassionate approach to feelings

CFT strategies often seek to cultivate feelings of warmth, courage, kindness and connectedness as a way to meet painful moments in your life with soothing and centredness rather than fighting them (and inflaming them) or getting swept away with them (which could lead to more suffering and impulsive behaviours that you and those around you may come to regret).

Anger or sadness can also be compassionate. They can be in the service of alleviating or preventing suffering. For example, feeling sadness at the plight of an unhoused family can spur action to help alleviate that suffering. Likewise, feeling enraged at racism and or social injustice, if used effectively, can lead to taking steps to advocating for change.

Sensory experiencing
As discussed, CFT (and ACT) encourages you to face difficult feelings rather than engage in unhelpful types of emotional avoidance. Being able to turn towards while bringing soothing to your sensory experience of suffering (e.g. pounding heart, lightheadedness) is like wearing a cosy rain jacket while stuck in a pouring rain storm. In CFT this begins with soothing rhythm breathing. Then it adds strategies such as mindful awareness of senses, training in bringing a warm and kind tone to how you talk to yourself (versus the punitive, harsh inner critic), and compassionate body postures to bring soothing and centredness when facing intensely painful moments.

The three targets (flows) of compassion

According to CFT there are three ways in which compassion can flow. Compassion can flow from us to others. Think about how readily you can care for friends, family and even a little lost child. Think about the compassion you would experience if someone you care deeply about had a serious problem, such as their home burning down. You would bend over backwards to be kind and helpful.

The next flow of compassion is allowing compassion to flow from others to yourself. This can be more challenging for many of us. Most people find giving compassion far easier than receiving it, though some of the more narcissistic members of the human species excel at receiving compassion from others but are uninterested in feeling or showing compassion to others.

Finally, the third flow of compassion is directing compassion towards yourself. Many people recoil at the thought of self-compassion. This used to be difficult for me. But think about it pragmatically. Think about the person you will spend the most time with in your life. Perhaps a romantic partner, a close friend or a sibling. The amount of time you will spend with that person will be a mere trifling compared to the amount of time you will spend with you. If you have a harsh, critical relationship with the one person you will spend 100 percent of your life with, then life will be much more difficult than it has to be.

The case for being self-compassionate

Human life is difficult and compassion can help.

The uncomfortable reality is that all humans, even famous TV psychologists, rich and famous celebrities, spiritual leaders and gurus, suffer. This book is not about how to never suffer, but how to meet suffering in ways that ease rather than inflame it — and compassion is a big part of that.

Why is human life so difficult?

THE MINDFUL FREAK-OUT

We freak out about things other animals freak out about

A zebra will have an intense threat reaction when it comes face to face with a menacing lion. We are no different. We get those same threat reactions when facing danger that is real and imminent. Just like them, when in danger we'll fight if we think we can overcome the threat. In the case of threats we know we can't overpower (lions, tigers and bears — oh hell no!), just like other animals our threat systems will convince us to run or hide. And just like a dog that lies on its back in a submissive posture in the face of a dominant attacker, we also have an appeasement instinct when it feels necessary.

Unfortunately, even in the modern world, with its walls, locks and other safety devices we've created, the world can still be a very dangerous place at times. Our threat systems, after all these years of evolution and development, are still important for our survival. However, just like my dog freaking out when he hears a dog barking on TV, our threat systems, because they are designed to be 'better safe-than-sorry' machines, frequently get triggered by false alarms.

> *Greg is walking down the street when a car backfires. He freezes and scans for danger as his heart pounds wildly in his chest!*

> *Jinny is hiking with her kids when she suddenly stops and swings her arms wildly to push her children behind her, protecting them from the 'snake' that upon further inspection she sees is only a stick!*

> *Anya screams suddenly when the 'ferocious spider' jumps on her leg — but it turns out to be fuzz that fell off a blanket!*

And we freak out about things other animals can't freak out about
Let's say you have a cute little pet poodle; we'll call her Sprinkles. While you are inside your home, Sprinkles is in your backyard. Suddenly, a large bulldog pushes the gate open and wanders into the backyard. Sprinkles is suddenly *very* upset. She growls and barks as Spike the bulldog plays with her toys and chews on her bones. She is as upset as a pet poodle named Sprinkles could possibly get. Then Spike's owner calls loudly for him and he runs off, leaving poor Sprinkles in peace. In a few short moments, Sprinkles is no longer upset. Her blood pressure and heart rate have returned to normal. You call her in for dinner and she happily runs in and eats. All is right with her world.

Now, imagine that Spike's burly owner, Mike (a bulldog of a man), whom you've never met, suddenly walks into your home. He turns on your TV and goes and makes himself a sandwich. He then walks around your house, eating your food, opens up the cupboards and rifles around your drawers and closets. You are rightly very upset at Mike. You may threaten him, hide from him, scream at him, and soon, he leaves. Sprinkles' threat system went off-duty as soon as Spike left, but for you it's different, isn't it?

You will replay the intrusion in your mind, over and over. Your blood pressure may remain elevated for days as you ruminate over your encounter! You try to sleep at night, but you can't because your mind remembers Mike's intrusion and warns, 'What if he comes back!' Meanwhile, Sprinkles is sleeping peacefully through the night, blissfully unconcerned about Spike.

Humans suffer more than other animals because we can relive our most difficult and traumatic experiences over and over (and imagine an infinite variety of dark possibilities), brought up by our own always-active minds. For us, threats don't need to be external or real to freak us out. We can be visited by endless threats brought to us by our own minds and imaginations.

There are ancient parts to the human brain
Even though humans stand at the very pinnacle of the food chain, we retain parts of our brains that are relics from long ago, as we evolved over millions of years from much more primitive creatures. Paul Gilbert calls these parts of the brain our 'old brain'.[4] It is our old brain that is filled with emotions and animal mentalities such as tribalism, aggression, sexuality, competition, attachment and so on.

Brain 2.0: The new brain 'upgrade'
Long ago in our evolutionary history, parts of our distant ancestors' brains began to change. They began to develop the ability to complexly imagine, ruminate and solve problems using recollections from the past and imagining the future. They also developed the ability to speak and use language and symbols. Grogg could tell his buddy Trogg where he could find fresh water just by emitting sounds out of his mouth. And they developed a sense of self and an awareness of how they compared to others.

These complex cognitive adaptations were quite the game changer! We went from barely able to survive the harsh world of predators, ice ages, droughts and famines to mega-cities and iPhones in a relative blink of an eye.

These new brain abilities make up what Paul Gilbert calls our 'new brain'. It seems like a great thing, right? We are at the top of the food chain, we have art, culture and civilization. We can even drive a remote-control car around the surface of Mars.

Unfortunately, like so many good things in life, it has quite a downside.

Our old and new brains create trade-offs

What happens when our new brains and our old brains get together?

We retain our old brain motives. Some of which are good. We care for our young. We can have a motive to care for and protect people we perceive to be part of our 'tribe' (such as family, friends, colleagues, neighbours, community). However, we also have darker instincts, such as perceiving people outside our tribe as the 'other'. Like other animals, sometimes we play nice with the others and sometimes we have the impulse to treat them like our enemy.

We have an old brain instinct to care for and protect certain people, and our new brains allow us to develop hospitals to heal our sick and wounded, and schools and libraries to educate us. Yet our old brain's tribal instincts can kick in along with an instinct to dominate certain others. And our new brain allows us to develop concentration camps, torture chambers, slavery and nuclear warheads. For every Mother Teresa, Martin Luther King and Mahatma Gandhi, there is the potential for a Vladimir Putin, Joseph Stalin and Adolf Hitler.

You might be in a committed romantic relationship; however, when someone you find attractive enters your life (real or imagined) your old brain might give you a powerful impulse to mate with that person. And if someone treats you or your loved one rudely, your old brain might label them as the enemy and start giving you fantasies of how you could harm them.

On top of that, as the Buddha discovered for himself 2500 years ago, our new brains can be aware of and anticipate that our days here are limited (to around 25,000–30,000 days) and if we live long enough we will age, decline and die. No other animal on the planet is burdened by that terrible knowledge. If you are taking your beloved family pet to the vet to be euthanized, only you will suffer from that knowledge. Your pet will never have the slightest hint of existential angst.

And to top it all off, we self-aware humans can also suffer because of our instinct to compare ourselves to other humans.

'They make more money than me!'

'I wish I was tall like them!'

'That person is more attractive than me!'

'What if I don't measure up?'

You'll never see a rabbit awkwardly staring at its reflection and wondering, 'I wonder if I'm losing my hair — oh, what will the other bunnies think?'

Our old brains want to protect us from threats and our new brains can search our memories for threats ('What if the dog bites me, like when I was a child!'). And our new brains can and will anticipate countless threats — limited only by our powerful imaginations — for us to worry about ('What if there's a global pandemic and the world shuts down!!'). Our brains keep busy preparing us for threats that are only taking place in our minds. Our threat systems then try to take charge, often succeeding in placing us on autopilot and letting instinct drive our behaviours.

Is it any wonder that with these tricky brains we tend to freak out a lot?

Finding balance: The CFT Three-System Model of Emotion Regulation

According to CFT, emotion systems in humans evolved as a way to help us survive and thrive.[5] To explain this, we must travel back in time ...

> *Imagine you are test-driving a time machine. You decide to pop back in time 100,000 years to take a peek at our prehistoric past. While sitting in the machine, admiring the flora and fauna of way back then, you notice an enormous, sweet-smelling flower and have the idea to step off the machine, pick the flower and take it back as a souvenir. As rotten luck would have it, when you step off the time machine you accidentally hit a button on the control panel. By the time you pick the flower, poof, the machine returns to modern times sans passenger. You are stuck and will need to live out your life in this ancient and very dangerous time.*
>
> *Ever the optimist, you decide to make the best of the situation and begin pondering what you will need to make a go of this life. Just then you hear a ferocious roar unlike anything you have ever heard. You can tell it is a hungry predator so your top priority becomes clear: above all else, you need to avoid threats in a world filled with threats! You must not get eaten.*

For this, we have our evolved threat system. You realize that if you get eaten, nothing else about life in these times matters. Our threat system is the dominant emotion system. It has to be. If you are peacefully strolling along in a beautiful forest and an aggressive sabre-toothed tiger starts to charge, you need your threat system to take over and act

THE MINDFUL FREAK-OUT

quickly to flood you with stress hormones and distressing thoughts in order to give you the strength, energy and motivation to run like hell! It would not be very adaptive if you stopped to smell the roses.

The threat system brings with it unpleasant emotions like fear, anger and disgust. The focus is on protection and safety-seeking. Chemically, this system works by releasing stress hormones which energize the nervous system (we don't sleep well or at all while this system is screaming in the background). It motivates people to take immediate safety action such as fighting, fleeing, freezing or hiding, or perhaps appeasing. Even though these days our threat system often misperceives danger, too little activation of the threat system may lead us to taking foolish risks such as texting while driving or eating petrol station sushi.

The threat system is what will hijack you when you begin to freak out. It will make you lash out in anger or flee from anxiety-provoking situations. It will never ask for permission before it takes over and drives your mind and body in whichever direction it feels is best.

> *You burned a lot of calories running from that sabre-toothed predator. Soon you notice your stomach starts to rumble and groan. You realize that it is not enough to not get eaten – you must eat! You get very motivated to start foraging for berries and begin thinking of how you can sharpen a big stick to make a spear for hunting meat. And while you're at it, you will need to find water to drink, materials to build a shelter, and perhaps other resources you can use to trade with the local homo sapiens. You may even want to try your hand at prehistoric hooking up.*

Life is more than just avoiding hostile creatures and other threats; we also need to be able to accumulate resources, which are important to survival as well. For that we have a drive system. This system is all about wanting, pursuing, achieving and consuming. The emotions that may be seen when the drive system is active include joy, pleasure and excitement. The drive system can feel great — but it is about doing and achieving, not soothing and relaxing. If you win the mega-lottery today you'll likely be so excited that you won't sleep for days.

Too little activation of the drive system, however, makes it difficult to get out of bed and do something productive or fun. Too much activation, on the other hand, can make someone obsessive, workaholic, or Elon Musk. Billionaires in the news often do not seem to be satisfied with their vast resources. There seems to be an insatiable craving for more and more. This is an over-active drive system motivating their life choices.

> *It is getting dark. You are exhausted and terrified. It's been a long day! You've managed to hide from or outrun the various predators around you — for now. You even found a tree filled with enormous juicy figs. That temporarily perked up your spirits and re-energized you. But now you notice that you are so very alone, muscles aching, and greatly fatigued. All you want now is to feel safe and connected to a group of other humans. You need to find a community where you can live out your days. You need to be part of a tribe.*
>
> *You are in luck! A couple of hunters were out scavenging when your time machine popped into their territory. They have been silently following you, staying hidden and observing.*

THE MINDFUL FREAK-OUT

They have concluded that you are a god descended to Earth. They beckon you to follow them to where their tribe is located. The members of the tribe welcome you into the safety of the group. You feel wanted and cared for. And soon you begin to care for these people as well. You are given food, water and eventually you are provided a mate. In the evenings you sit around the fire and take in the beauty and kindness of your new family. You are loved and in return you feel love for them. You feel safe in your tribe – and a kind of peace you never felt before. You are home.

There are times when our brains perceive that there is no immediate threat and there is nothing we need to go out and acquire at the moment. In those times a third emotion regulation system can kick in. This one is called the soothing or safeness system. This is associated with feelings of peace and contentment. When this system predominates, we feel safe and that our needs are met, for now. This system involves an increase in calming neurochemicals such as oxytocin and the activation of the parasympathetic nervous system, which helps us feel safe and soothed.

Our soothing systems evolved to be responsive to kindness, warmth and caring. After a strenuous day of hunting and gathering, our ancestors would return to the relative comfort and safety of the tribe, where they could 'rest and digest'. They did not have to come home from work only to be faced with isolation, bills, taxes, action movies on TV, horrific news stories from people around the world, and social media FOMO. How times have changed.

CFT uses a variety of strategies to access our soothing systems so that we can find balance in lives where we routinely encounter stressors (threat system) and often live over-scheduled, overachieving lives (drive system). This allows us to rest and recover and is often fuelled by cultivating positive relationships (with others and ourselves) that help us feel caring and cared for. By waking up the soothing systems when feeling overwhelmed by painful emotions, we can feel more grounded in the moment, disengage autopilot, and then gain a wiser, calmer perspective on which action will serve us best.

Think about it this way. At times, we will all experience intensely painful emotions related to our threat systems. Whether someone has stolen a parking space we had been waiting for, or we are having an anxiety attack due to a phobic trigger, our threat systems *will* try to take over and direct our behaviours. If we can get off autopilot then we have a choice. We can throw gasoline on the emotional fire by acting based on our threat-instincts (even when it runs counter to our value system) or we can actively work to wake up our safeness systems in order to ground ourselves so we can choose a values-based response to the situation. The goal of the safeness system isn't emotional avoidance, but to get in touch with the centredness, wisdom, strength, courage and caring needed to face a difficult moment.

KEY POINTS

- Being human is very challenging at times – all of us suffer.
- Compassion seeks to address suffering using two skill sets.

THE MINDFUL FREAK-OUT

- The first skill set focuses on becoming *aware* when we or others are suffering (rather than being stuck on autopilot).

- The second skill set is focused on *preventing and alleviating* suffering.

- Increasing compassion for others and ourselves is related to many physical and mental health benefits – and it can be intentionally cultivated.

- A compassionate mind is one that is strong, wise and committed to helping.

- We all have an innate soothing system that is associated with calm, peaceful feelings. This system can help balance out our threat and drive systems.

7

COMPASSIONATE MIND TRAINING

You may have had the experience of having an argument with a loved one, when suddenly you feel under threat and defensive. This person in front of you who you love is suddenly being perceived as your antagonist. Then, you become aware of the pain you can see in their eyes — perhaps they begin to cry. Suddenly, like waking from a nightmare, you once again see them as your loved one and you see that they are suffering. *Then* you are able to look for a mutual resolution to this disagreement. You are no longer interested in defeating them.

This is compassion in action. And wouldn't it be great to wake up much earlier from the nightmare of needing to defeat an opponent? Perhaps the opponent you see is your own thoughts or painful feelings, and you begin to struggle with yourself. When you are at war with someone you love, who is going to 'win'? When you are at war with yourself (and your own emotions) who is going to 'lose'?

THE MINDFUL FREAK-OUT

When in the midst of a highly distressing moment, once you are off autopilot you can use a compassion-focused strategy to get centred, stop the war and bring your Best Self to face the moment. For some this will come naturally and for others compassion will need to be trained in order to receive its benefits. This training, detailed in this chapter, is like going to the gym to build up your compassion muscles. As with any exercise, consistency is the key. Ideally, you would try each of the exercises and practise at least one to two of them each day. Some of them, you will learn, can be integrated into your daily routine. Some can be quite short whereas others may take longer (perhaps 10 minutes, give or take).

The following compassionate mind training exercises are adapted from the CFT literature.[1]

Shifting attention towards compassion

With compassionate awareness, you practised waking up to the present moment using mindfulness and helpful intentions. Now that you are off autopilot, you can take a step further into shifting into a compassionate mindset to bring online a sense of inner strength, wisdom and a commitment to alleviating suffering. This is all in the service of responding to life's painful moments in a way that is consistent with who you would like to be.

To learn to shift from a threat focus to a compassion focus, it helps to practise consciously directing your attention. Try this quick attention shifting exercise:

- **Notice your right foot. Pay attention to it for 10 seconds.**

- **Now shift your attention to your left hand. Pay attention to it for 10 seconds.**
- **Now spend 10 seconds with your attention shifted to what you can hear.**
- **Now notice for 10 seconds everything you can feel with your body.**

Good. Now what did you notice about attention? If you are like most people, you noticed that you could fairly easily shift your attention from one thing to the next, at least for a moment. This isn't perfect. Most likely your attention got pulled all over the place. But you were likely able to direct it where you wanted.

What happened when you focused on your right foot? It's likely you noticed more details about it and could feel sensations in and around it. What happened to your right foot when you shifted your attention to other targets? Likely it was cast into shadows within your mind and attention. Your foot didn't go away; you were simply less aware of it and more aware of other things.

When you are stuck in your threat system, compassion often gets cast into the shadows. By shifting your attention back to compassion, even a little bit, you shine a spotlight on the parts of you that are helpful and balancing when you feel out of control. This can activate the safeness system so that you feel less under threat. The more you practise shifting into your compassionate mindset the easier access you'll have to it.

There are many exercises you can use to strengthen your compassionate mind. Here is a collection of them.

Compassion-focused imagery

Imagery is the mental pictures and movies playing in your mind. Some people can get perfectionistic when it comes to imagery exercises, thinking their images should come in high-definition clarity. It seldom works that way for most of us. It is okay for images to be fleeting and shifting; just do your best to bring your attention back to the images when they fade or you become distracted.

You might think you cannot make images in your mind. If that is you, ask yourself, 'What is a bicycle? How does a rose smell? What does pizza taste like? What is the sound of frying bacon? What does it feel like to hold an ice cube?' When doing this, it's likely your mind gave you at least vague impressions of each of your five senses. Please be compassionate with yourself if these images are imperfect — it is common.

Try all the exercises below and practise the ones that seem like a good fit. If they all feel awkward it may be that this is just a very different sort of practice than you are accustomed to, and you might become more comfortable with them over time. You might have a deeper reluctance to experience compassion for a number of reasons. If that is the case, check out Chapter 14, 'Fears, blocks and resistances to compassion'.

You will notice that each of the exercises begins with centring yourself using your breathing. This is advised in CFT as a way to make optimal use of the exercises.

Compassionate colour

- Find a comfortable place to sit. Close your eyes if that is comfortable.
- Use soothing rhythm breathing to centre yourself.
- It can help to adopt a body posture and facial expression

that represents warmth, strength, wisdom and deep commitment to caring.
- Now select a colour that represents warmth and kindness for you.
- Imagine that colour is a pleasant mist or light that flows around and through you.
- Imagine that within this colour are the attributes of strength, wisdom and a commitment to easing any suffering you are experiencing.
- Imagine this colour is there to build you up — to support you.

You can do this exercise for as long as you like. Perhaps practise it for only 30 seconds when you are experiencing a difficult moment, or find a more peaceful time to do this for 5 or 10 minutes.

Safe place imagery
- Get comfortable and begin with a couple minutes of soothing rhythm breathing. Allow your eyes to close if that feels okay for you.
- Bring to mind the type of place that for you might bring up feelings of peacefulness and contentment — a place that feels safe. It could be a place you have been to in the past, a place you have seen on TV, a place you have read about, or an ideal place existing only in your imagination.
- Imagine your sensory experience of this place. What do you see, hear, feel and smell?

THE MINDFUL FREAK-OUT

- Imagine that this place has an awareness of you — it welcomes you and wants you to feel at ease.
- You can choose whether to imagine you are alone in this place or with comforting people of your choice.
- You also can choose what you are doing while there; perhaps you are sitting and just soaking it all in.
- Spend as much time here as you would like before coming back to the present.

Keep in mind that for this exercise you are bringing up a place where you feel safe and peaceful, rather than a place representing physical safety. For example, you might be safely locked in a bank vault with twelve ninjas as bodyguards and a massive gun in your hand pointed at the entrance to the vault — that might be a safe place, but it is likely tied into your threat system instead of your soothing system.

Metta (loving-kindness) meditation
I think of the metta meditation as being a thorough workout for the compassion system. It is an ancient form of meditation that has been studied extensively in recent decades and has been shown to decrease suffering and increase wellbeing.[2] Parts of the exercise might be a bit difficult as it includes self-compassion and compassion for someone you find difficult. Other parts will likely come more easily.

- Find a comfortable place to sit. Allow your eyes to close if that feels okay. Begin with a couple of minutes of soothing rhythm breathing.
- For this exercise, you will be asked to imagine different

people. For each person you will say the following words in your mind with a warm and gentle tone as you focus on your intent to offer compassion to that person:
- 'May [person's name]_____ be happy.'
- 'May _____ be free from suffering.'
- 'May _____ be free from harm.'

- Let's start with bringing to mind someone you care about — someone important to you. Focus on the intent to feel warmth and kindness along with well-wishes towards them as you say the above phrases in your mind, beginning with, 'May _____ be happy.'
- Next, think about someone on the periphery of your life, someone you see regularly (like a neighbour, coworker or your child's teacher) but are not close with. Repeat the phrases with warmth and with a desire to feel well-wishes towards them (it's okay if you don't feel it).
- Now think about well-wishes for yourself. With equal warmth say the phrases, but change them to 'I' ('May I be happy …').
- This time, think about someone you find a bit difficult. Repeat the phrases with warmth and the wisdom to realize that even this person suffers and is doing the best they can given their upbringing, genetics and multitude of life experiences that they didn't choose.
- Finally, consider how difficult human life can be and send well-wishes to all people everywhere, using the phrases 'May all people be happy …'.

What did you notice?

Feel free to tailor the phrases in a way that is personally meaningful for you. Perhaps, for example, you might wish good health or freedom from pain. If you find it feels too unpleasant to send well-wishes to a difficult person, feel free to either select a less triggering person or to persist, noticing that it can become less challenging over time.

Compassionate memories

In the same way that a vivid memory of eating a delicious slice of pizza triggers your body to produce saliva, bringing up compassionate images, like memories, has the potential to activate the physical and mental health benefits of bringing your soothing system online.

MEMORY: COMPASSION FLOWING TO YOU
- Find a comfortable seat and let your eyes close or stare at a blank space on the floor or wall in front of you. Begin with a couple of minutes of soothing rhythm breathing.
- Now, recall a time when someone was warm, caring and kind towards you. Try to recall a time that felt supportive and soothing, but not one where you were in a lot of distress.
- Try to recall the person's kind facial expression and body language as they showed you kindness and support.
- Bring to mind the caring tone in their voice.
- Recall how it felt to receive this kindness.
- Take a moment and savour the warmth of this memory, allowing yourself to feel gratitude towards this person.

Allow your face to adopt a kind expression towards this person.
- When you are ready, slowly return to the present moment.

MEMORY: COMPASSION FLOWING TO ANOTHER
- Find a comfortable seat and let your eyes close or stare at a blank space on the floor or wall in front of you. Begin with a couple of minutes of soothing rhythm breathing.
- This time, recall a time when you were kind, warm and caring towards another who was struggling or suffering. This could be a person or perhaps a pet. Try to pick a memory where you felt a sense of inner strength or authority, were wise in not judging the one who was struggling, and were committed to being helpful.
- Try to recall your sensory experience of that time. Remember what the situation looked, sounded and felt like.
- Recall the gentle sound of your voice as it was directed in a soothing way. Recall how your compassion was reflected in your facial expression and body movements.
- Focus on what being compassionate in that moment felt like throughout your body. See if you can soak that in now.
- As you let the memory fade and return to the present moment, see if you can carry those compassionate qualities with you as you go about your day.

THE MINDFUL FREAK-OUT

Using memory to access a compassionate mindset can be a simple, readily available strategy when you find yourself struggling with an emotionally painful moment. Try to select memories that were positive experiences of caring or being cared for, rather than ones where you or another was experiencing intense distress.

Ideal compassionate other
In this next exercise, you are invited to create your greatest inner ally: your ideal compassionate other.

- Find a comfortable seat and let your eyes close or stare at a blank space on the floor or wall in front of you. Begin with a couple of minutes of soothing rhythm breathing.
- In the privacy of your own mind, consider the qualities you would like in an ideal compassionate other.
- This other can be a person from your life, or someone fictional like Albus Dumbledore. It does not need to be a person, though: it can be a spiritual figure or force, it could be an animal, or some cosmic entity straight from your imagination.
- Your compassionate other is wise. They know that we have 'tricky brains' and that so many of the difficulties we experience are not of our design and are not our fault.
- Your ideal compassionate other is filled with inner strength and a sense of courage and authority. They are there to share their strength with you.
- And they are committed to caring for you

— unconditionally. They are on your side and are there to help, however they can, to support you and ease any suffering you may be experiencing.
- Consider how you would like them to appear to you. Their height, age, gender and other characteristics. Notice how they express their compassion to you in their tone of voice and in their facial expressions and body language.
- You can choose to sit back and bask in their compassionate presence or ask for help or support about something that is causing you distress, and then soak up their wise guidance.
- You can spend as much time here with your ideal compassionate other as you would like, before you come back to the present moment and carry this support with you throughout your day.

If your mind jumps around from image to image, that is normal and okay. You might find that over time you settle on an image or two that you most prefer. Or you can have a team of compassionate others who are looking out for you in times of distress or just when you need a bit of soothing.

You can combine your ideal compassionate other with your safe-place imagery to have an ideal meeting spot for your ideal source of support.

Acting like your ideal compassionate self
- Imagine you have been cast to star in a movie. In this

movie you play yourself, but a version of yourself that is your ideal of compassion — towards yourself and others. This ideal you is filled with a deep sense of courage, confidence and inner strength. They are also wise. They know that human life can be difficult and we all are doing the best we can with the cards we were dealt — and we didn't choose those cards. This is the wisdom of non-judgment.

- Your ideal compassionate self has a deep commitment to caring for yourself and others. This self is motivated to ease suffering. They know that life will present challenges and they strive to find a compassionate way to deal with these challenges.
- Now it is time to get into character. Think about how the ideal compassionate version of you would sit — perhaps keeping your spine straight, shoulders back and head stacked over your shoulders. Try to embody this version of you using your posture. Then, allow yourself to adopt the facial expression for this role.
- Imagine you are performing as your ideal compassionate self. How do you relate to other people, those you care about, those you encounter day to day, and perhaps people who you find challenging? How would this version of you move through the world? How would they solve problems that came their way?
- Now allow your eyes to close or stare at something neutral. Allow yourself to get centred by focusing on your soothing rhythm breathing for 30 seconds.

- Imagine you can see that ideal compassionate version of you as if you are looking at another person. Notice how they are dressed. Notice their facial expression and body language. See their sense of inner strength, wisdom and kindness radiating from them.
- Imagine walking up to them and stepping into this image and becoming one with it, feeling those compassionate attributes throughout your body and mind.
- When you are ready, open your eyes and come back into the room, and bring those compassionate attributes with you into your day.

It is okay if you do not *feel* these attributes. If you don't, continue to practise acting as if you had those attributes while being open to feeling what you can. Can you embody your compassionate ideal self when you are driving, riding the bus or dealing with a situation at work? See if over time you can add more opportunities to be your compassionate ideal.

Befriending yourself

Many people I encounter have a difficult time with the concept of intentionally being self-compassionate. Yet they are usually eager to provide compassion to others in need. Though they might at first struggle with accepting compassion from others, it is nothing like the struggle against being kind and supportive to themselves.

If you find the idea of self-compassion uncomfortable or even repulsive, please see Chapter 14, 'Fears, blocks, and resistances to compassion'.

THE MINDFUL FREAK-OUT

If you are open to exploring self-compassion further, please read on.

Being self-compassionate when you are in distress is like having an inner ally or close friend with you, supporting you. While harsh self-criticism makes a difficult moment worse, self-compassion during a difficult moment can help soothe the savage beast within us. You know this instinctually. When a loved one is in distress, do you criticize and berate them? Of course not. You speak to them in a warm, gentle and kind manner. You attempt to be helpful.

It is sad that while we find it natural to bring compassion to others, we often treat ourselves with harsh cruelty during our most challenging moments.

Let's change that pattern — starting right now. You *are* worth it.

Compassion for the freaked-out self

Let's practise bringing compassion to yourself during a difficult moment.

- Find a comfortable seat and let your eyes close or stare at a blank space on the floor or wall in front of you. Begin with a couple of minutes of soothing rhythm breathing.
- Think about your ideal compassionate self. Remember the attributes of inner strength and courage, and hold your body posture in such a way (sitting upright, shoulders back, chin slightly lifted). Imagine being filled with these attributes, and along with them the wisdom to not judge and the commitment to being caring and helpful.
- Bring to mind a time that was difficult for you. This could be a time when you were faced with a moment of high anxiety, tremendous anger or deep despair. For the

first few times you practise this, select a time that felt somewhat difficult but not overwhelming.
- Now imagine that as your ideal compassionate self you visit the *you* who was suffering in that difficult moment. Imagine you can go back in time to that moment with the intent to lend support to the *you* who was suffering. Only that other *you* can see or hear you.
- Notice the suffering they are experiencing as you try to be as helpful as you can. Imagine what you would do. Consider how your tone of voice would be towards that *you* and how your body language would communicate your caring intent.
- Offer any kind and encouraging words or helpful behaviours to this *you*, treating them like someone you care deeply about.
- When you are ready, come back to the present moment in this room and proceed with your day with the intention of continuing this caring and supportive stance towards yourself.

Self-compassion using your image

Another way to practise offering yourself compassion is when you see your image in a mirror, during an online video meeting, or when looking at a photo of yourself. Sadly, so many people look at their image in a judgmental, perfectionistic and critical way. Actor Paul Giamatti demonstrates this in the movie *American Splendor* where he plays self-critical comic book artist Harvey Pekar. Harvey is shown walking by a mirror, catching his reflection and cringing while he says, 'Well, there's a reliable disappointment!'

The 'radical' notion here is to build yourself up rather than tearing yourself down. Try this when you see your reflection or image:

- Take a breath and resist the urge to criticize yourself.
- Instead, see yourself from the outside. From a wise, strong and caring perspective. See this person as a worthy human being who has struggles — like everyone else. And they are, like all of us, trying to live the best life they can while dealing with the tremendous challenges of being human.
- Offer yourself a kind smile and (at least in your mind) some words of encouragement.

It is okay if this is difficult and you are not feeling it at first. This can be a challenge. Stick with an intention of wanting to feel compassion for yourself. Over time what begins as an intention may (like the ending scene in the movie *Casablanca*) be the start of a beautiful friendship.

Compassionate behaviour practice

If you practise being compassionate in the course of your day-to-day life, it will be much less difficult to access compassion during your most challenging moments. Set an intention to begin to treat yourself in the way you would like a compassionate other to treat you, or the way you would like to treat others whom you care deeply about.

Practise acts of self-compassion:

- Take the time to make or acquire a favourite food for dinner when you are having a difficult day.

- Kindly speak out for what you would like to do this weekend, rather than keeping silent and agreeing to what another wants.
- Take a bubble bath — just because.
- Get a massage.
- Say 'no thanks' to something that is asked of you when you feel over-committed.
- Prioritize self-care such as exercise, sleep, rest, leisure and caring for your health.
- Get yourself a gift you would like to receive (for example, flowers).

And you can practise acts of compassion for others:
- Give your partner flowers, a massage, or a big hug or a compliment — not just on special occasions.
- Tell a friend how much you value their friendship.
- Give compliments to people you know and those you encounter — find something you admire about them and tell them.
- Give a friendly smile to people you walk by, especially if they seem like they could use one.
- Hold the door for the person behind you — let them enter the building first.
- In the supermarket, let the person with only a few items ahead of you in line when you have a full basket.
- Call an old friend you have not spoken to in a while. Show an interest in how they are doing.

By building practices like these into your life you keep your compassion pump primed and ready for when you (or those around you) need it the most.

The golden rule of compassionate behaviour

You know the golden rule: treat others the way you would want to be treated. Good advice, right?

There is a different golden rule when it comes to compassion: treat yourself the way you would treat a close friend or loved one in that situation.

It can be very difficult for some of us to wrap our head around the concept of being self-compassionate. When going through a difficult moment, our inner critic shows up just in time to kick us when we are down. If that happens to you, you can lean on the golden rule of compassionate behaviour.

- Take some time to imagine how you would treat a cherished person in your life if they were going through a difficult time. What would your tone of voice and your body language be like?
- What would you advise them to do about their challenging circumstances? Would you advise that they react impulsively based on their threat system alarms? Or would you help them slow down and talk it out, using a soothing tone and encouraging words?
- Direct the same care and consideration towards yourself that you would give to them.

Even though you might not *feel* you deserve the same consideration, logically you can understand that you are compassionate with people you care about because you know it is more helpful than tearing them down. Therefore, even if you don't feel it, it makes sense to do what is most helpful for you when you are in distress. Kicking yourself in your darkest moments won't help you or anyone else muster the inner strength, wisdom and commitment needed to alleviate suffering and move through a difficult moment.

KEY POINTS

- Compassion helps you bring your Best Self to face distressing moments with inner strength, wisdom and a caring commitment.

- Compassionate mind training is designed to build your compassion muscles – and consistency is key.

- Engaging your compassionate mind begins with intentionally shifting your attention towards a compassionate focus. For example, using imagery, meditation, memories and your image.

- Acting as your compassionate ideal and engaging in intentional compassionate behaviour practices helps prime your compassion system to be available to you when you need it the most.

Once you have shifted into a more compassionate mindset, you can use that sense of inner strength, wisdom and caring commitment as you

THE MINDFUL FREAK-OUT

turn to face your own emotional distress. The next step is to let go of the struggle against your inner experience.

8

NOTICING AND RELEASING STRUGGLE

Can you remember a time when you were stressed out, but because you were so caught up inside your own head you didn't realize it until much later? At the end of the day, perhaps you noticed a headache, stomach discomfort or general muscle tension and realized, 'I've been really stressed out today!'

Have you noticed what you do with your body when feeling emotionally distressed? You likely tighten your muscles (whether you are aware of it or not) in reaction to the painful feelings. We do this in the same way we might tense up when having painful dental work — it hurts, we don't like it and we automatically brace against it.

White knuckling against uncomfortable experiences, however, increases suffering during those moments. As legendary Swiss psychiatrist Carl Jung said, 'What you resist not only persists, but will grow in size'. And, as the compassion researcher Kristen Neff says, 'Suffering = pain x resistance'.[1]

Rather than inflaming painful emotions by resisting or struggling with them we can actually decrease suffering by practising radical acceptance. In addition, facing your emotions without struggle gives you more freedom to move towards what is important in your life.

Here are a couple of metaphors that help drive this point home and encourage release from emotional struggle.

Getting stuck in emotional quicksand

One of my favourite ACT metaphors is that of quicksand. You have likely seen on TV or in movies where an unsuspecting traveller finds themselves in the unfortunate position of stepping into quicksand — and the more they struggle the faster they sink.

Imagine that an intense emotion you are experiencing is like quicksand. You were just going about your day when suddenly … splash! You've just fallen in. You don't want to be pulled under where you are sure to drown in that sandy, sludgy mess. Your instinct kicks in and you automatically begin to struggle, kicking and flailing, desperately trying to propel yourself out of this mess. This makes you sink more. The prospect of dying in this way is terrifying so you flail around even harder, fighting with all your might to free yourself … and you sink even further.

What you are doing *feels* like it should be working, but it's making matters worse. You pause for a moment, take a few breaths. You realize that struggling makes you sink faster , so you decide to try something different. You stop struggling and spread your arms and legs out and float with the quicksand. You try to contact as much of the surface area of the quicksand as you can. It is scary for a moment as you let go of struggle, but then you notice something — you've stopped sinking.

When we are feeling strong, painful emotions we naturally want to fight and struggle with them. Why do we do this? We are often taught to try to fight our emotions from a very young age. Think of the frustrated parent who tells their crying child to 'Stop crying or I'll give you something to cry about!' On top of that we humans have an unfortunate habit of comparing how we feel on the inside to how happy and peaceful others appear in their social media pictures. We do this, forgetting that the image posted does not reflect the reality of a person's actual emotional life. So when we feel distressed, we are naturally tempted to fight to feel the way we think we should feel — often with opposite results!

The struggle switch

Writer and ACT trainer Dr Russ Harris has a clever metaphor for the perils of struggling with painful emotions. He calls it the struggle switch.[2] It goes like this …

It seems like we all have a struggle switch in the back of our minds. When a painful feeling shows up — as painful feelings do for all of us — we feel uncomfortable. In the face of this discomfort the struggle switch can get turned on. When anxiety shows up and that switch gets flipped, we tend to fight and struggle against the anxiety. This serves to give us anxiety about our anxiety — and cranks up suffering. Seeing this, we might then experience even more anxiety about the fact that we are anxious about our anxiety.

Then we can get so fed up that we begin to feel frustrated about our anxiety! 'I hate this anxiety! Why do I have to feel this? It's not right!' Then perhaps sadness joins the 'party'. 'I can't believe this is my life. It's never going to get better. Why bother?' Then enters guilt. 'I can't believe I am feeling sorry for myself when there are starving children in the world.'

What started as anxiety gets amplified through struggle. Other emotions jump in and soon we are preoccupied and less open to the world around us; it can even pull us into self-defeating behaviours. It is tempting, though, to struggle to end painful emotions — they're painful! However, we must ask ourselves, has all the fighting and struggling to rid ourselves of painful emotions succeeded in setting us free from painful emotions? It hasn't.

What if we can flip the struggle switch back to *off*? Then there we are with the anxiety, an uncomfortable emotion we all experience. But rather than fighting and struggling with it, we can make space for it and allow it to ease in its own time. Meanwhile, we can refocus on doing those things in life that are important to us.

Now let's practise turning off your struggle switch.

SKILL BUILDING: MINDFUL BODY SCAN

> For the next few moments I invite you to practise letting go of the struggle against emotion. At the outset, this might seem like a relaxation exercise, but that is not what it is. This practice is about softening into the emotions rather than struggling to change or eradicate them.

- You can practise this with your eyes open or closed, seated, lying down, or even while standing in line at the grocery store. You can choose to begin with a couple of minutes of soothing rhythm breathing if time permits.
- Now we are going to focus on different muscle groups. The goal is to notice where you are gripping, bracing, struggling or fidgeting. These behaviours often relate to struggling against the emotion you are feeling. The goal then is to let go of the struggle as much as you are able. If you are tightening, loosen. If you are moving or fidgeting, allow your muscles to soften as much as they are willing. Your emotion might change or it might stay the same, but it is not something you are trying to control — you are trying to let go of struggle and control.
- Start with your feet. Notice tightening or fidgeting. Now see if you can let go. Let whatever you feel remain for now and see what it is like to not struggle against it. Now move to your calves and shins. Let go of struggle. Notice tensing or bracing in or around your upper legs and hips. Let go of struggle. Notice if your stomach muscles are tensing, even a little. If so, allow them to soften as much as they are willing. Notice your fingers, hands, wrists and forearms. See if they are tensing or fidgeting in any way. If so, invite them to soften the struggle. Allow yourself to fully feel, with gentleness, whatever there is to be felt. Do the same with your upper arms, biceps and triceps. Notice your lower back, and up through your upper back and shoulder blades. Soften struggle where you find it. Notice if your shoulders

are tight or bunched up. If so, allow them to soften as much as they are willing. Let yourself feel what you feel — openly and willingly. Now pay attention to your neck, inviting any strain to ease. See if your teeth and jaw are clenched together, even slightly. Invite them to soften, making space for your emotions to be there with gentle permission. Do the same with the small muscles around your eyes, forehead and scalp. Let go as you settle into your emotions rather than strain against them. Notice if there are any other areas of struggle against emotion and allow those areas to let go as much as they are willing.

You can spend as much or as little time as you want on this exercise. If you have time and privacy, this can be a longer exercise. If you have neither the time nor privacy (if you are giving a talk at work, for example) you can pause, ever so briefly, and do a 1- to 2-second mental check-in with your body and catch and release struggle as you find it. Over time, you might find you carry your struggle in a specific predictable area. Perhaps you tighten your stomach, or maybe you grit your teeth. If this is the case, you can check in very briefly with those specific target areas only, given time constraints.

Below is another technique for letting go of struggle, which focuses on the breath. I encourage you to try it and see how it works for you. Again, the idea is not to try to turn this into an emotion control strategy; we're not trying to oust anger or exterminate anxiety. Rather, this is another strategy for making as much peace as you can with painful emotions rather than inflaming them through struggle.

SKILL BUILDING:
BREATHING OUT STRUGGLE

> Like the previous exercise, you can practise this with eyes open or closed, sitting, lying down, or out in the 'real world' such as while hanging out with friends at a social gathering.

- Begin by finding your soothing rhythm of breathing.
- Now with each inhale focus on *breathing in the emotion*, feeling it fully and gently.
- With each exhale, focus on *breathing out the struggle against the emotion*.
- Inhale, open to the feeling. Exhale, surrender the struggle, softening into the emotion.
- Repeat for several minutes or as long as you prefer.

KEY POINTS

- You increase your suffering when you fight against your painful emotions.
- This struggle is often automatic and outside your awareness.
- Intentionally noticing and releasing the struggle during a difficult moment can ease suffering.

Now that you've made some space for the distressing feelings that have shown up, let's turn our attention to the threat-based thoughts that are accompanying the feelings.

9

UNHOOKING FROM UNHELPFUL THOUGHTS

As you let go of struggling with your painful feelings, you might notice that your mind remains noisy. Thoughts, mental images and memories are a mental 'all-you-can-think' buffet that never ends. The question is, which thought items will you put on your plate and consume with your attention and actions?

Not all thoughts are useful. In fact, with our better-safe-than-sorry threat-sensitive brains, very often our thoughts are unhelpful noise:

- 'I'm not attractive enough!'
- 'People won't like me!'
- 'I can't do anything right!'
- 'The plane is going to crash!'
- 'I can't tolerate these feelings!'

THE MINDFUL FREAK-OUT

The never-ending thought buffet is always open and always tempting us to consume more and more. Here is the 'little secret' that Acceptance and Commitment Therapy wants you to know: you don't have to consume the thoughts that naturally show up for you. While we have zero control over the types of thoughts that swirl around in our minds, we can take steps to avoid hooking onto unhelpful thoughts. Or, if we are already hooked, we can take steps to unhook from them.

In ACT this process is called 'defusion'. Rather than being fused with the thought (e.g. 'The plane is going down') we can defuse (unhook) from this unhelpful thought. It is the process of stepping back from thoughts, getting distance from them, and seeing them merely as mental noise. This gives you the space to decide if you wish to act on them or just let them pass.

> *Sasha is driving home on the highway after a long and stressful day at work. The traffic gets tight and suddenly it is bumper to bumper. Her mind yells to her, 'You're trapped!' With that thought she grips the wheel tightly and tenses her body. Her anxiety increases. 'You're going to have a panic attack – you'll lose control of the car and your body! You better pull over or else!' Noticing those thoughts, Sasha begins to fight her anxiety in an attempt to avert 'disaster'. This makes her anxiety worse and then her mind tells her, 'You better pull over or something really bad will happen!' Sasha immediately complies and pulls off the road into a carpark. She is fusing with her disaster thoughts and treating them as if they are true.*

Mindful acceptance of thoughts

A helpful way to learn to defuse from unhelpful thoughts is to practise mindful acceptance of thoughts. This ACT strategy involves learning to see thoughts as thoughts rather than judging them or hooking onto unhelpful ones. This is similar to the other mindfulness strategies we have practised, but instead of focusing on your breath, your senses or emotions without judgment, we are focusing on thoughts.

The idea is to recognize that your brain is a mental noise maker and to learn to see what pops into your mind as a thought rather than a fact or something to run from, struggle against or actively try to get rid of. If the thought is not helpful then you don't need to attach to it.

Let's take the thought, 'Going out is a bad idea — I'd better stay at home'. Imagine, like most people would, you are feeling quite anxious when starting your new dream job. That thought pops into your head as you are ready to head to work on your first day. This thought can make calling in sick tempting. You might try to get rid of the thought only to notice it doesn't go away — in fact it gets louder. You try to make yourself think only happy thoughts while struggling to clear your mind of this less desirable thought. Only you can't rid yourself of a thought by trying to make it stop. That only makes the thought more present in your mind.[1]

Try this

Reader, it is of vital importance that you *do not* think about eating pizza. Don't do it! Don't think about that hot, cheesy, delicious pizza. Don't think about how it looks, how it tastes, or that wonderful aroma of a freshly baked pizza, made just the way you like it. Rid your mind of all pizza-related thoughts.

Set a timer for 60 seconds and every time you have a pizza thought, make a mark on a sheet of paper.

On your mark, get set, go: get rid of pizza thoughts now!

What did you notice? If you are like most, you likely found that pizza thoughts were more present in your brain when you tried to not think about them, not less. Trying harder to get rid of them just made more thoughts bubble up to the surface.

Thoughts can be helpful or unhelpful, depending on the context

Thoughts aren't always unhelpful, though. Some will be useful to hook onto, depending on the context. Let's take the exact same thought from earlier: 'Going out is a bad idea — I'd better stay at home'. This time, however, the context is different. Instead of needing to go to work, you have a final exam tomorrow that you are unprepared for. It is Saturday night and your friends are texting you, pleading with you to meet them at a bar for a late-night booze-fest. In this case, this same thought is helpful if you value your education and future career. Hooking onto this thought (and thereby staying home to study) moves you closer to your valued goals and away from the gut impulse to procrastinate.

It is not always easy. Our thoughts can be powerfully seductive.

Bruce's marriage is on the rocks. His spouse is fed up with his drinking and, frankly, Bruce is sick of the hangovers and feeling ashamed of his behaviour. There is nothing more important to him than his marriage so he hasn't taken a drink in a week. He is determined to repair his relationship and his health.

Today, however, has really tested that resolve. His boss got on his case for something that wasn't Bruce's fault. Then his car broke down on the highway in the pouring rain on the way home from work. When he reached for his phone to call for help, he realized he'd left it at the office. Then he gets home 3 hours late only to have his spouse accuse him of going to the bar with friends after work.

'Just take a drink,' his mind encourages, 'just one little drink.'

The next thing he knows, Bruce is going to the liquor cabinet and he starts to reach for the gin bottle. 'Have that drink, you deserve it,' his mind tells him. Bruce pauses for a moment. He recognizes that powerful urge to drink. He notices he is having a thought that he should have a drink. He takes a few slow breaths and reminds himself how important his marriage is to him and that he wants to improve his relationship with his spouse, and his health. He makes a choice to not hook onto the thought and urge to drink. He is determined to choose his own path rather than be at the mercy of his thoughts. He turns away from the bottle and towards healing his marriage.

Unhooking from the multitude of seductive but unhelpful thoughts can help put you back in the driver's seat of your own life.

Awareness of thoughts

We don't choose our thoughts. Swarms of them fly through our minds with the slightest of provocations. I invite you to practise noticing your thoughts that automatically show up. I'll show you some words and

THE MINDFUL FREAK-OUT

notice what naturally happens in your mind.

Read these words and then pay attention to the thoughts that come up:

- Parents.
- Work.
- Politics.

See how easily a variety of thoughts get activated in your mind — notice how automatic it is. We don't get to control the fact that thoughts are popping into our minds all the time. The challenge is to avoid hooking onto those that are unhelpful.

> *Tina hates her job. Who wouldn't, given how abusive her supervisor has been. Tina longs to find another job, but the thought 'I'm not smart enough to start over at a new job' has led her to give up on finding a better job. She is remaining at a job she hates. She feels stuck.*

Tina could benefit from defusing from her thought, 'I'm not smart enough'. At the same time, however, she could allow herself to hook onto a more helpful thought — 'It's time to start looking for a job' — and decide that attaching to this thought and taking action based on it (searching for a new job) could serve her well in alleviating her daily suffering at work.

Let's learn how to defuse from unhelpful thoughts.

SKILL BUILDING: DEFUSION FROM THOUGHTS

Take a moment and notice the thoughts flowing through your mind right now. When one pulls at your attention, say in your mind, 'I'm having the thought [fill in your thought here]' and let go of it (For example, 'I'm having the thought "I'm not smart enough"').

Now let's try it again, but this time when a thought pulls at your attention say in your mind, 'I'm aware that I'm having the thought [fill in your thought here]' (for example, 'I'm aware that I'm having the thought "I'm not smart enough"').

There are a number of variations of this defusion approach that you can utilize when distressing thoughts show up:

- 'I'm aware that my brain is giving me the thought "I'm not smart enough".'
- 'There's that "not smart" thought again.'
- 'Oh, there's that old familiar thought again.'
- 'Thanks for the thought, mind. I know you're trying to help in your own way.'

What was that like for you? For some, it is very challenging. That's okay. As with anything else, practice will build this skill over time. Remember to use a kind inner tone when learning a new skill.

THE MINDFUL FREAK-OUT

ACT defusion metaphors

ACT uses a range of metaphors to aid in defusion. This section will present you with various defusion metaphors adapted from the ACT literature. I encourage you to try them all on and see which approaches feel useful to you. Use only those that you find helpful.

The mind as a glitchy helper

Even when we feel tormented by our thoughts, our minds are trying to help — in their glitchy sorts of ways. For example, in the case of Tina, whose mind warns her not to look for a better job because she's 'not smart enough', her mind wants to protect her from what *it* perceives to be a threat. By convincing her she's not smart enough, her mind is trying to keep her with what is familiar and 'safe'. Remember, throughout most of human history we were hunter-gatherers. The unknown was far more undesirable than a predictable source of food and water. Even now, our minds often crave what is stable and predictable.

In my last book, I used the metaphor of **the anxiety beast**.[2] This was inspired by the fairy tale Beauty and the Beast where, at the beginning, it appears that the Beast is the villain of the story, tormenting others with villainous glee. Later in the story, we come to learn that the Beast, while very rough around the edges, is actually a well-intended hero. Our threat emotions, like anxiety and anger, are like that: on the surface they may look and feel scary, but at their core, these emotions are trying in their glitchy way to keep us safe. They rush in to protect us from what they perceive (or misperceive) to be threats.

When you notice unhelpful thoughts popping up (e.g. 'Don't do it — you're not smart enough!') imagine your very own goofy, kind-hearted 'beast' jumping up and down in front of you trying to help. You can even respond with a 'Thanks for trying to help, big guy, but I got this'.

Another favourite of mine is thinking of your threat-thoughts as coming from your inner **guard dog**. Your guard dog is your very own fiercely loyal, hyperactive and overzealous inner protector. It is always on the lookout for whatever may be a threat. It barks about you being late to an appointment. It barks to warn you to call your doctor if it thinks you are seriously ill. It may look into the future and bark about emotional devastation when you consider asking someone on a date. Our goofy guard dogs mean well, but they are still dogs. No matter how well you train them, they will never be anything other than dogs. Our threat systems will always be imperfect protectors.

When you are experiencing highly distressing thoughts, you can take a step back and remember that your mind is not trying to torment you, your inner labradoodle is just howling — most likely at shadows. You can imagine petting your guard poodle while waiting for it to eventually lose interest and move on to something else.

Another glitchy helper metaphor is the **toddler sheriff**. Imagine a tiny toddler wearing a sheriff's costume along with their nappy. I imagine mine as having squirt guns in their holster and a big plastic sheriff's badge pinned loosely on their vest and way too big sunglasses hanging crooked on their face. The Toddler Sheriff's job is to serve and protect, whether we want it to or not. When feeling under threat, you can imagine that nappied dude rushing to rescue you, but he has the reasoning abilities of a two-year-old. 'Thanks, little dude, but I got this.'

Nature defusion metaphors

Nature metaphors are popular mindfulness approaches to help get distance from unpleasant thoughts. Here are some of my favourite ones for

THE MINDFUL FREAK-OUT

practising unhooking from thoughts.

Leaves on a stream: Take notice of your thoughts as if they are written on colourful leaves floating down a beautiful stream on a pleasant autumn day. You can sit on the soft grassy bank and watch the leaves come, and watch them go. They move at their own pace.

You might catch yourself at times splashing through the water, trying to clear the stream of the leaves. That is what trying to get rid of your thoughts is like. It's futile, however, as more leaves come and after a while you get exhausted with the impossible task. Alternatively, you might jump into the water and grasp at the leaves, holding them up to your eyes, examining them over and over. While you do this, however, you are missing the beautiful day around you — examining one after another in an endless loop.

You have a choice. You can stay in the water and ponder the writing on the many leaves or struggle to clear the stream, *or* you can climb out. You can settle back onto that comfortable spot on the bank of the stream and return to watching those colourful leaves just float on by, in their own time.

Ocean waves: It's a sunny summer day and you are lounging at the beach. You are sitting, watching and listening to the waves come and go. Each wave represents a difficult thought. They come in and they go back out. No need for you to do anything other than watch them rise and fall and return.

However, you might find yourself fed up with the waves and want them gone. They are noisy, after all! You march down the beach, into the water, and push at the waves falling into you. You try in vain to hold back raging thoughts. Yet they continue to crash into and around you no matter how hard you try to fight them off.

It is an exhausting battle. Instead, you can come out of the turbulent water and settle back onto the beach. You can once again relax as you watch the waves from a distance.

Waterfall: You find yourself standing under a powerful waterfall. The waterfall represents the chaos that is the constant deluge of human thoughts. They are pounding down on you. It is impossible to see what's around you. The noise is ear-splitting — you can't hear anything beyond the roar. While under this waterfall, you can focus on nothing else — you can do nothing other than try to stay upright as the unrelenting weight pushes you down.

You can choose to either stay put or move forward step by step. You move forward, and suddenly you emerge and look around to find yourself in a beautiful clearing. You step out of the water and turn to watch the waterfall of your thoughts showering down as you relax on the shore. From a distance you can even admire the beauty of the waterfall — without it holding you down. You can watch your thoughts without being pushed around by them.

Thunderstorm: Our thoughts are like the weather — we can't control them. Some days are sunny and mild, but others can be stormy. We don't get to pick the weather, and hating storms does not make them pass any quicker. When your mind is storming with unpleasant thoughts, images or memories, you can notice it and then choose to calmly carry on with life knowing that the storm will pass in its own time. The more we rail against the reality of the storm (whether mental or meteorological) the more we suffer. Instead, you can imagine staying in with a hot cup of tea and watching the storm do its thing out in the distance.

THE MINDFUL FREAK-OUT

Other defusion metaphors

Beach ball in the pool: You head over to the pool for a relaxing swim. It's a nice day outside and as you get in the pool you find that the water is pleasantly warm. As luck would have it, you have the pool to yourself. In this metaphor, your distressing thoughts are a large inflatable beach ball that has blown into the pool and smacked you in the head.

What do you do?

Unfortunately, in this metaphor the ball must remain in the pool. So you attempt to rid yourself of this annoyance by shoving it underwater. But, as you do so, it immediately springs back up and bops you in the face. Now you're determined. You shove and shove, but the ball violently pops back out of the water each and every time. The ball will never go away by sheer effort.

You can decide to let the ball (your thoughts) be there in the pool with you as you go about your swim. Occasionally it still makes contact with you, but mostly it floats around the pool all on its own. Your arms, legs and attention are now freed up for you to finish your swim.

Other people's children on the plane: As a parent of three, I remember those days of taking babies and toddlers on airplanes to visit Grandma. These are not peaceful memories. One would cry, two would bicker, and all three would whine and climb all over the seats. And I remember the annoyed looks of the other passengers as we would board with three children, three child seats, and an overstuffed bag of snacks, nappies and distractions. I could almost hear them praying in their minds, 'Please don't let them sit next to me'.

Imagine you are one of the lucky passengers who did not have to sit next to us. Instead, you can relax in your seat and watch a movie, read a book, get some work done or perhaps chat with the person next to you.

Unhooking from unhelpful thoughts

In this metaphor, the young children are seated six rows behind, with their parents. They represent your distressing thoughts, images or memories. They can be noisy at times, even though they aren't right next to you. *But you are not the struggling parent.* You don't have to feed them, entertain them or change their poopy nappies. It's not your responsibility to quieten them. They can be annoying, but they are doing what young kids do on long plane rides.

Let the parents handle it while you turn your attention back to flying how you want to fly. Watch that movie or chat with your neighbour. You can even pat yourself on the back knowing that with all its discomforts, rather than avoiding the journey towards your desired destination you chose to brave the unpleasantness in the service of living based on what is important to you (visiting family, furthering your career, or taking a well-earned vacation).

After a while, you might even notice that the children have fallen asleep. The turbulent thoughts eventually subside.

Speaking of children, here is one more defusion strategy that uses very young and tiny humans. I like the child metaphors because they allow us to bring compassion into the mix.

Preschool teacher: Imagine you are a preschool teacher. You are the authority in a room filled with rambunctious two-year-olds. The children are running around doing and saying silly, childish things, as they tend to do. You have the wisdom to understand that they have newly developing brains that make them irrational, impulsive and emotional. Your job is to care for these little goofballs, not to judge them, debate them or obey their childish demands.

Among the chaotic crowd of feisty toddlers you notice Suzy Sadness, Andy Anxiety and Amy Anger. They all have something to say and they

THE MINDFUL FREAK-OUT

all have their own wants. Suzy Sadness may tell you to withdraw from activity, Andy Anxiety may try to convince the class to play hide and not seek and Amy Anger just yells and wants you to help her smash things. All the children want to tell you how to teach *your* class!

But you are the teacher. You can retain a sense of wisdom, caring and authority while letting the children babble on. You can pat them on the heads and thank them for their suggestions, but you are the one who gets to decide what the class does and focuses on. The thoughts in your mind can yell and demand, but you get to decide how you want to be in your life.

The variety of defusion strategies is limitless. They all work towards the same goal: loosening your attachment to the noise your mind makes so that you are not automatically reacting to it. Rather, you are able to take a moment and consider how you would like to respond. Think about the episodes of air-rage that have ended with adults being forcefully removed from the airplane while they tantrum like toddlers. In those moments they are fused with a thought such as 'No one can tell me what to do — I'll show them!' In those moments, those thoughts and the threat system they are attached to have taken over that person.

KEY POINTS

- We can't control the types of thoughts that pop into our minds.

- Many of the thoughts that enter our minds are unhelpful; they do not move us in a valued direction.

- We can avoid hooking onto these unhelpful thoughts (or get unhooked) using defusion strategies.

Now that you have learned to get off of autopilot and used your compassionate mind to help you face a distressing moment, it is time to take valued and compassionate action.

PART 3

RESPONDING BASED ON YOUR BEST SELF

(Compassionate Action)

10

NOTICING AND NAMING URGES

As we have discussed, your emotions — especially threat emotions — can take over and make you act on impulse. Unfortunately, there are very real risks to responding to threat emotions impulsively, as many residents of prisons and visitors to divorce attorney's offices can attest to. Our goal, therefore, is to make our own choices, preferably from the perspective of our Best Selves.

This can be difficult, to say the least!

Remember, the same emotions that pull out all the stops trying to save you from the hungry bear chasing you are the same ones that can show up for you in safe situations, such as when you're having an argument with your spouse or getting ready to give a talk at work.

If a bear is chasing you, then your threat system is giving you a hand by triggering a powerful urge to act quickly and defensively. However, when you are having a disagreement with a loved one, reacting quickly and defensively can take you far away from what is important to you

THE MINDFUL FREAK-OUT

— caring and connecting with your loved one. Have you ever 'won' an argument only to injure a relationship? Have you ever avoided something that is important to you (like social opportunities) because anxiety talked you out of it? Threat emotions can give you strong impulses that can pull you away from living based on what is important to you.

So far, you have learned strategies for regaining control (getting off autopilot) when threat impulses seek to lead you astray. Then, you practised ways to turn and face challenging situations from a compassionate mindset. In the following chapters you will learn how to act based on your Best Self.

The first step is to recognize what your threat emotions are urging you to do.

An urge *will* emerge!

Urges are impulses that just show up — whether you want them or not. Some urges are good. When our bodies need food or fluids, it is desirable to have an urge to eat or drink. When a child is hurt or lost, most people have an urge to help. And if we consider doing something that is dangerously reckless, such as climbing a massive mountain wall with zero safety gear (such as Alex Honnold's 2017 free-solo climb of El Capitan in Yosemite National Park) most of us would have a powerful urge to pick another hobby.

And then there are other urges that, while normal, aren't so helpful:

- **The urge to text your old flame when you've just had a disagreement with your current one.**
- **The urge to escape into alcohol, chocolate or Netflix**

- **whenever contemplating leaving an abusive relationship.**
- **The urge to smack your teen who just told you where you can stick your chore list.**
- **The urge to avoid facing a fear that stands between you and the life you want.**

Some urges can be so subtle that you may not even realize you are acting on them. Such as the urge to tense your muscles when you feel stressed. Or to hold your breath or breathe shallowly when anxious. Or to ruminate over a perceived wrong.

Other urges are less subtle. For example, the urge to scream when riding a terrifying roller-coaster or the urge to quit your job when your abusive boss publicly berates you.

Our different emotions can lead to different types of urges. Anxiety often leads to urges to avoid a perceived or misperceived threat. Anger leads to urges to lash out. Sadness leads to urges to withdraw from people and activities. And affiliative feelings such as warmth, caring and love lead to urges to assist, protect and connect. The specific urges (what to avoid, who to lash out at) vary from person to person. One may have the urge to give a rude cashier the stink eye while another may feel pulled to violence.

What is important to understand is that these urges are automatic. They were created for you, not by you. You cannot choose the type of urges you have, nor their intensity. However, if you are aware of them (if you are off autopilot) then you have a better chance to override them and choose your own desired response to a difficult situation.

THE MINDFUL FREAK-OUT

Roy's boss is giving him a hard time. After all, he was only 5 minutes late. Yet he has been receiving a stern rebuke for the last 10 minutes. He is feeling his blood boil listening to his boss go on and on about irresponsibility. He was fired from his last job for getting into a shouting match with his former boss. However, he can't lose this job — his family is counting on him. He lets go of clenching his fists, slows his breathing, and sits more softly in his chair. He recognizes that he is angry and notices that he has a powerful urge to yell at his boss. He decides to make space for his anger, allowing it to rise and fall without giving in to expelling the emotion physically or verbally at his boss. He notices that the anger begins to recede over time. He gets to keep this job.

Urges can lead to hasty attempts at quick fixes. Sometimes, giving in to it might pay off, but you are gambling on autopilot to make the best decision about your long-term wellbeing during highly distressing moments. It is like gambling on a hyperactive two-year-old to make life decisions for you during difficult times.

SKILL BUILDING:
MINDFUL AWARENESS OF URGES

> Stopping to notice your urges during highly distressing moments is challenging. As with most things, practice can help. In this exercise you will recall a difficult moment and mindfully notice which urges emerge. This exercise was

Noticing and naming urges

  adapted from CFT's multiple selves exercise.
- It is helpful to begin mindful exercises with a minute or two of soothing rhythm breathing.
- Now, let's go on an exploratory mission to see which urges your emotions offer up for you. To do this, think of a situation that is mildly to moderately distressing for you — something that wakes up your threat emotions. For example, recall a recent argument with your romantic partner. Now let's check in to notice which urges or impulses show up for you.
- First, let's notice the anxious part of you. Try to see the world through the eyes of your anxiety. Where do you feel it in your body? What kinds of thoughts, images and memories does it bring into your mind? Notice how your body automatically reacts to the anxiety, perhaps by tightening your muscles or altering your breathing. Now see if you can observe what your anxiety urges you to do about the distressing situation. You don't have to agree with the urge, but simply see that it is something that shows up (for you, not by you). Give the urges a descriptive, non-judgmental name, for example 'I am noticing there is an "urge to avoid"'.
- Now go back to focusing on your breathing for 30 seconds to help you re-centre.
- This time, let's notice the part of you that feels sad about the distressing situation — even a little bit. Where is it showing up in your body? Notice what types of thoughts, images and memories spring up around this feeling. Is your

THE MINDFUL FREAK-OUT

- body reacting differently to the sad part? See if you can notice what urges the sad part presents to you. Give those urges names. For example, 'Here is an "urge to isolate from others"'. See if you can watch and hold gently these urges, without acting on them.
- Go back to your breathing one more time for 30 seconds.
- Now, let's see if you can notice the angry or irritable part of you that shows up when you recall the distressing situation. Do you experience it in different parts of the body than for the other two emotions? Notice the thoughts, images and memories that show up for the angry/irritable part of you. Notice how you respond to the emotion (with openness or resistance?). Now, notice what urges the angry side of you pulls you towards. Give them a name. For example, 'Here is the "urge to get revenge".' Watch the urges as if you are a scientist watching microbes in a microscope — with gentle curiosity.
- Return one last time to the breath for 30 seconds, and when you are ready, open your eyes and come back to the room.

When you are in an emotionally distressing moment, use your growing mindfulness skills to notice and name your immediate urges. Observe those powerful unhelpful urges when they try to take hold of you. Then, rather than giving in to the unhelpful urges, learn to surf them.

Urge surfing is a mindfulness strategy designed to enable people to withstand unhelpful urges.[1] It involves the mindful acceptance of urges, which enhances your ability to choose an alternate behaviour instead of automatically giving in to urges.[2]

SKILL BUILDING:
URGE SURFING

- Allow yourself to get into a comfortable position. Take a few centring breaths and then let's begin.
- Notice an urge you are experiencing right now. It could be a desire to scratch an itch. Or perhaps you notice an urge to move part of your body. Maybe you are hungry and have an urge to eat. Or maybe this feels boring and you have the urge to rescue yourself from this exercise with a phone distraction.
- Once you've selected the urge, find where you feel it the most in your body. What do the sensations feel like? How much space does it take up in your body? Is there a colour associated with the urge? Notice whether there is a texture associated with the urge. Notice if the urge feels like a steady pressure or involves tingling sensations.
- Urges are like waves. They rise, they crest, and they fall — in their own time. Imagine that your urge is an ocean wave. It builds and rises, gathering strength and size. Watch it grow. Use your breath to 'surf' the wave. Breathe in the urge and breathe out the impulse to distract, push away or struggle with the urge. If your mind wanders, that's okay. Bring your attention back to the urge in your body.
- Like an ocean wave, notice your urge rise, crest and fall. Other waves may follow, and you can surf those as well. Some waves are bigger and more powerful, and others less so.
- Notice that you can be present with your urge without being washed away with it.

THE MINDFUL FREAK-OUT

Try to practise urge surfing in your daily life. Are there important goals you have, like losing weight for health reasons? Surf the urge to grab that bag of chips. Do you have the urge to make your work or school report perfect, but just need to get it done? Surf the urge to check it one more time. Want to stop checking your phone compulsively? Surf the urge to turn away from work to watch another cute cat video.

KEY POINTS

- We are often driven by urges that we may not even be aware of.
- You can learn to check in to notice what urges are present.
- Then, rather than giving into them you can learn to surf your urges.

Now that you have explored the emotions and urges that show up for you around a distressing situation you are in a better position to decide whether to act on them or not. Now is the time to choose how you want to respond to an emotionally painful moment.

11

CHOOSING YOUR BEST SELF RESPONSE

No one is immune to moments of high emotional pain in life. In this chapter we are going to consider some painful moments you have experienced and try to answer these questions:

- How have you responded to these situations in the past?
- What was the short-term outcome?
- And what was the long-term outcome?

We will consider what those responses have cost you (or how they have benefitted you) in terms of suffering, impact on your relationships and the pursuit of what is important to you. Did those responses move you closer or further away from the life you want to live? Often, what feels better in the short term causes more problems in the long term.

THE MINDFUL FREAK-OUT

Let's look at some examples:

Distressing situation	How I responded	Short-term outcome	Long-term outcome	Did it move me closer or farther from the life I want?
My doctor asked me to come in to discuss my blood test results.	I cancelled my evening plans, stayed home and Googled symptoms, trying to figure out what was wrong.	Relief to cancel plans, then much higher anxiety as Dr Google said I was dying!	Worse anxiety, plus I missed out on being with friends, and feel bad about myself for going down the Google rabbit hole.	Further away! I don't want to let anxiety keep me from connecting with my friends.
Disagreement with my spouse over chores.	I raised my voice and called her a slob.	I felt better for a moment having vented, but she was hurt and angry – and the chores were still not done.	We are having worse marital problems. Not sure we will make it. Me pushing her made her less likely to help around the house.	Further away. If we get divorced, then I am completely on my own for chores and general support.
Invited to a party.	I accepted the invitation even though I was very anxious about it.	I was worried ahead of time and uncomfortable at the start of the party. It felt easier over time.	I am making new friends, starting to date, and I am getting more comfortable socializing.	Closer. It was hard at first, but so worth it!
Driver cut me off in traffic.	I drove close behind them and continued to honk the horn. Then I pulled alongside, rolled down my window and yelled at her!	I felt like I was in the right and was teaching her a lesson!	I felt angry for the next few days. My family saw me acting horribly and don't want to ride with me when I am driving.	Further away. My daughter will be driving soon and I would hate for someone to treat her in a threatening way. Also, I hate feeling out of control like that!

Choosing your Best Self response

Your turn. Describe some recent distressing situations, how you responded, and what the outcome was:

Distressing situation	How I responded	Short-term outcome	Long-term outcome	Did it move me closer or farther from the life I want?

THE MINDFUL FREAK-OUT

What is your Best Self?

Let's review where we are so far in facing an emotionally distressing moment. You've worked hard to disengage your autopilot and mindfully ground yourself in the present moment with a more compassionate mindset. You have noticed and named what your emotions are demanding of you. And now it is time to choose how to respond to the distressing situation.

You have a choice between reacting to a situation based on threat emotion or responding based on your 'Best Self'. I am defining Best Self not based on how you feel (i.e. 'If I feel happy I am my Best Self'). How you feel is often out of your control. Behaving based on your Best Self means making choices based on your deepest values. These values reflect who you want to be in your time on this planet. Additionally, your Best Self seeks to ease or prevent suffering. As we've discussed, easing and preventing suffering in the long term often means turning towards what is difficult or painful (like facing a fear or studying for final exams) in the short term.

In other words, taking action based on your Best Self involves values-based compassionate responding.

Defining your values

Values are chosen qualities of how you want to behave in the world.[1] For example, you might value being:

- **adventurous**
- **kind**
- **courageous**

- **honest**
- **humble**
- **loving**
- **patient**
- **spiritual**
- **productive**
- **and of course, compassionate.**

What is your heart's deepest desire for how you want to be with others and with yourself? What type of friend or parent do you value being? What do you value with respect to your health and wellbeing? When you aren't sure what to do, values are like beacons in a thick fog, illuminating the direction to move towards.

There are a few important points about values. First, values are a direction, not a destination. Let's say that one of your top values is family. If you set a goal of visiting your parents over the holidays, that's a fine goal to have based on your value of family. However, you can't declare victory and check family permanently off your to-do list. If you are living your value, then you will create more goals to regularly reflect that value.

Second, values are freely chosen. You might have a lot of 'shoulds' that show up when you think about your values:

- 'I should accumulate wealth and power!'
- 'I should be more adventurous!'
- 'I should value romance!'

It's important to let go of the shoulds and open up to what you truly want your life to stand for. If you are living based on your values, you are setting goals that are inherently rewarding to you.

Finally, feelings are not values. Saying, 'My top value is feeling happy' is disempowering as you often can't control how you feel. Values are destinations you can move towards with your body — and it bears repeating, values are a direction, not a destination.

Who do you want to be when the going gets tough?

Think about times you've experienced highly distressing moments in your life. There were likely times when you behaved in ways you can feel good about. Perhaps you paused before sending a rage-text and decided to sleep on it only to see things differently in the morning.

However, like all of us, you've likely had times when you've reacted to such situations in ways that you later regretted. Perhaps you fled an anxious situation and missed out on an important moment in your life. Or perhaps you've ranted and raved at someone using colourful language and hand gestures as a commentary on their driving skills.

We've all been there. We've all been hijacked by threat emotions in difficult moments. And we have all done things in the heat of the moment that we later regret. In 2019, Pope Francis was shaking hands with admirers in a crowd. One woman, in awe of meeting him, was overzealously holding his hand, fervently caught up in the moment. The Pope's autopilot took over and he slapped her. He later apologized for his behaviour, which ran counter to his values.

The fundamental question is: once you get off autopilot and have the freedom to choose how to respond to challenging moments, how do you want to respond? If you were at your best, your wisest, calmest, most caring and confident, how would you want to respond now and in the future to difficult emotional and interpersonal situations?

- **Anxiety will give you the urge to avoid.**
- **Anger will give you the urge to strike out.**
- **Sadness will give you the urge to withdraw.**

However, these are not laws or commandments that you need to follow. If you are off autopilot, you can override these primitive signals bubbling up from the deep recesses of your brain.

We can feel anger at someone and choose the path of peace. We can feel anxious in a situation and choose to march forward. And we can feel sad and reach out. We can be psychologically flexible during difficult moments.

So, back to the fundamental question in this chapter: Who do you want to be when the going gets tough?

THE MINDFUL FREAK-OUT

SKILL BUILDING:
VALUES CLARIFICATION – TOMBSTONE EXERCISE

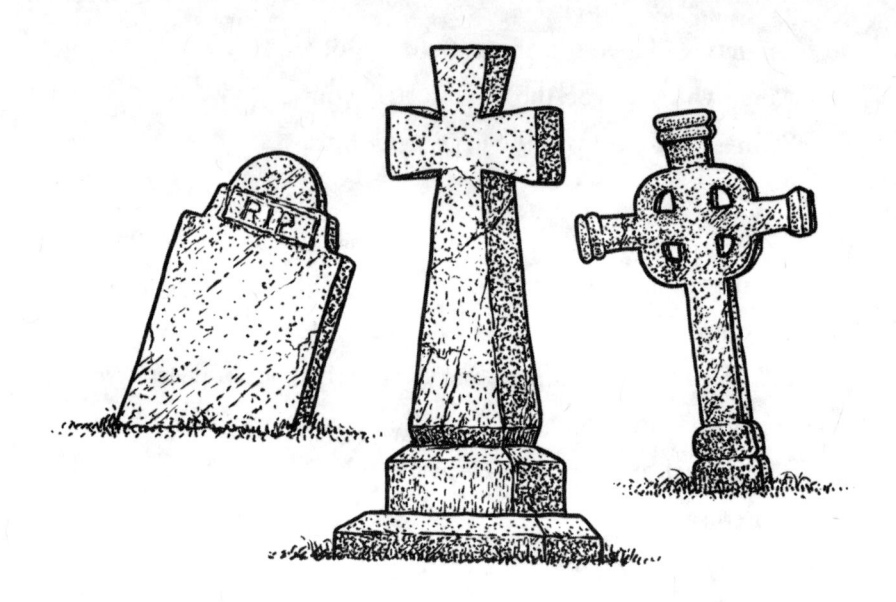

ACT values exercises often cut to the heart of what's important. No more so than the simple, yet profound tombstone exercise. Let's try it.

Take a look at the tombstone above. It is a reminder that human life is finite. None of us is here much longer than the average of 25,000 to 30,000 days we get. Then our earthly ride comes to an end. Look at the image of the tombstone above; what do you want yours to say about you? Take a moment and really think about this. Do you want the essence of your life to say:

- 'I won petty arguments with my spouse, friends and random drivers'
- 'I avoided doing things that increased my anxiety'
- 'I kept my life as comfortable (and non-eventful) as possible'
- 'I stayed away from new people and situations to avoid discomfort'?

What do you want your brief time on this planet to stand for? Take a piece of paper and write what you want the message on your tombstone to say about you and your life. Write a brief sentence or two that sums up how you want to be remembered.
What you write down says a lot about what is truly most important to you.

Other ACT values clarification exercises:

A well-lived life

Take some time to ponder the following:

Imagine you have had a long and well-lived life. You are coming to the end of your days and you are reflecting upon your life and accomplishments. What are you most proud of? What and who in your life was most important to you? In what ways did you handle life's challenges that you feel good about as you look back?

Now take some time and write your reflections on a sheet of paper. What themes can you spot?

I know these exercises are a bit morbid, but I believe there is nothing more powerful than the awareness of our mortality to focus us on what is absolutely most important. On that note, how about we add one more such exercise?

My Final Years values clarification exercise
Imagine you are meeting with your doctor following some tests. Your doctor walks in and says, 'I have some bad news and some good news for you. I'll start with the bad news. The bad news is that you have five years to live. At the end of five years, your body will give out. The good news is that you will feel fantastic for the next five years. You will feel energetic and healthy. You will also feel confident and all the old insecurities and self-doubts will be gone. You will be the absolute best version of you until the peaceful and painless end.'

- On a sheet a paper, record your answers to the following questions: How would you spend those last five years?
- Who will be important to you and how will you treat them? Remember, this is the absolute best version of who you could be.
- What will be important for you to do during this time?

See if you can find a theme within your writings and ponderings that pertains to some of life's important domains such as:

- **work or education**
- **leisure time**
- **relationships**

- **personal development (spiritual, health or other personal growth values).**

You can tweak this exercise by imagining the doctor gives you one year to live, or one month, or only 24 hours. If you had one last day, would you spend it trying to settle scores and win arguments? Would you scream at the driver who cut you off? Or would you take the opportunity to forgive and connect deeply with the important people in your life? Would you stress over being perfect in some way, or would you cut yourself a whole lot of slack?

There are many books written on developing a lifestyle based upon your deepest values. This is a core focus of ACT. For this book, however, we are now focusing on a specific aspect of values. That is, if you were living your deepest values of who you truly want to be, how would you want to behave when life brings you highly distressing moments and suffering?

Sticking with your values during highly distressing moments

Suyin has a phobia of driving. During the first two years of Covid she was able to work from home, which made her fear worse because she no longer needed to deal with her fear by making the 30-minute drive to her office. Now even the thought of getting behind the wheel is enough to trigger a powerful panic attack. She relies on her spouse to drive her and their three-month-old baby anywhere they need to go.

Now her worst nightmare is coming true. Her spouse is away on business and their daughter has just developed a high fever. Suyin just got off the phone with the pediatrician, who wants her to bring the baby to the clinic right away.

Suyin is highly anxious at the prospect of getting behind the wheel again. However, she is willing to experience any panic attack her nervous system can generate if it means she can take care of her precious child. She loads the baby into the car and takes off for the clinic. Along the way she vows to do whatever it takes to overcome her phobia.

I saw a video recently of a belligerent, intoxicated man accosting a large mixed martial arts champion in a supermarket carpark. The smaller man was pushing the champ in the chest and raising his fists challenging him. The champ stood his ground while talking gently, asking the man if he was okay and if he needed some help. The smaller man could see kindness in the champ's eyes and began to cry. The champ gave him a hug and the smaller man hugged him back.

This was a distressing moment that could have turned out very poorly for the intoxicated man, but the champ was in touch with his Best Self and acted in a way that was consistent with who he wanted to be in the world.

Take a moment and consider this: who do you want to be when distressing situations arise (and they will arise, as they do for all of us)? Imagine you are being awarded a lifetime achievement award late in your life. The person presenting the award is talking about your life. At one point the presenter says, '... and they handled adversity by _____.'

If you were behaving like the absolute best version of you, how would you want to respond when:

- conflict arises
- plans change unexpectedly
- painful thoughts bubble up
- anxiety-provoking situations present themselves
- life brings crushing disappointment
- you feel rejected by another
- difficult emotions take hold
- you or someone you love is diagnosed with a life-threatening illness?

There is no right or wrong answer. It comes down to what is in your heart. Who do you want to be when things are going well *and* when life gets difficult? It can be helpful to bring to mind (with self-compassion, not self-judgment) a time when you responded to a challenging moment in a way that, in hindsight, you don't feel good about. If you are like me, you have a lifetime dotted with such times. If you could go back in time, with the benefit of greater wisdom, empowerment and a commitment to caring for yourself and others, how would you advise the younger you to handle the situation?

Likewise, can you recall a time when you handled a challenging moment in a way you felt good about? It's okay if you can't think of anything. You get to move forward from here newly committed to a more values-based way of responding to difficult moments.

Who are your distressing moment role-models?

Another way of clarifying who you want to be during life's challenging moments is to think about those you admire. Is there someone you have met in your life who handles emotionally painful moments in a way you would like to emulate? For me, it would have to be my grandfather, now long deceased. My grandfather approached life's challenges with grace, humour and respect. He was the first person to explain, in his folksy way, about the importance of getting off autopilot and responding to adversity in a thoughtful way. He used to tell me, 'When you lose your head, your ass goes with it.' Folksy, but it gets the point across.

Who in your life has been a positive role-model for dealing with challenges? What was their approach? Would that style be consistent with your values and be helpful for managing the challenges that come up in your life? If so, try these behaviours for yourself. If they are useful and you practise them repeatedly, they will become ingrained — and more available to you when difficult moments arise.

Not all of us, however, have had the benefit of a grandfather doling out old-timey wisdom. That's okay. How about a favourite character from TV, movies or books that you might wish to emulate? Which characters do you admire based on how they deal with adversity? Be careful not to confuse admiring how they deal with adversity with being entertained by how they deal with adversity. Way too many characters on the silver screen handle their adversity with guns, fists and vengeance — and usually escape the consequences of those actions.

My top movie role-models would have to be characters portrayed by Robin Williams, in both *Good Will Hunting* and *Dead Poets Society*. In both movies he comes across as a real person (not a superhero) who faces challenges, not always perfectly, but does his best to live his values when things get tough. Which behaviours from characters do you admire and would you want to borrow and try on to see if they fit?

How would you advise a loved one?
A compassion-focused strategy to help you decide how to respond to a distressing moment is to take yourself out of the situation (mentally) for a moment and imagine it is someone else facing this situation — someone that you care deeply about. How would you advise that person to handle the situation?

> *Zara's anxiety is trying to get her to stay home 'where it's safe', rather than going to the airport to catch that flight back east to visit her mum. The thought of getting on a plane is terrifying for her and she has a strong urge to cancel the flight. She hasn't seen her mum in a couple of years because of Covid, but now her mum's very ill and it feels important to go see her.*
>
> *Zara takes a moment and imagines it is her best friend who is in this situation. She takes a few breaths and imagines she is talking to her friend who is frightened to get on the plane. She realizes that while she would support her friend either way, she would encourage her to face her fear and get on the plane. Zara knows that her friend would suffer knowing she gave up the chance to see her mum, maybe for the last time. This gives Zara the perspective and motivation needed to get on the plane when her mind is telling her to avoid the flight.*

If you could have a do-over, what would you do differently?
We have all had those situations in life where we wish we would have handled things differently. So, if you could go back in time and do it all over again, how would you handle one of your highly distressing situations from the past? Imagine you are approaching it from a place of

greater wisdom, inner strength, and a dedication to easing suffering in the long term. Remember, this would be an action based on who you want to be and what you want to stand for.

It's all about workability!

In the end, the choice of how to respond in a difficult moment is all about the most important ACT concept: workability.

At the beginning of this chapter, we looked at the short- and long-term consequences of behaviours and whether the specific behaviours moved you closer or further away from living based on your values. If a behaviour moves you closer, it is workable. If it moves you further away, it is not workable.

Let's look at some examples.

When Shari and her spouse have a disagreement, Shari feels rage towards her spouse. This rage feels intensely uncomfortable, like she'll explode! When she feels this, she screams at her spouse, sometimes breaking things, and often storming out of the house while slamming the door shortly after calling her spouse a variety of four-letter epithets! Discharging her rage in that way makes her feel better in the moment, but leads to more fighting, heartache and shame later on.

In this example, Shari's behaviours help her feel a bit better in the moment, but lead to long-term suffering and a likely dissolution of her marriage. Additionally, when things settle down, she is mortified by her behaviour as it runs counter to her religious value system, which is an important part of her life.

It might initially be more uncomfortable for her to mindfully sit with those angry feelings while acting on her value of being a good listener and connecting with her spouse; however, in the long run she will get to live based on her values while decreasing the likelihood of the suffering she would experience from losing her relationship. By making space for her feelings, additional behaviour options can emerge, such as learning better communication skills by seeking out a couple's therapist or their pastor.

> *Carmelita has always been very socially anxious. She had thought that by her mid-thirties it would have gone away, but it has only intensified. Over the years she has avoided more and more social events. When she is invited to a party, she feels an intense wave of anxiety wash over her. She quickly comes up with an excuse to turn down the invitation, which brings her immediate relief, but each subsequent invitation brings even stronger anxiety. On top of that, outside of work she has become somewhat of a hermit – spending her evenings alone, less anxious, but with growing regret over missed friendship and romantic opportunities.*

Carmelita is hooked on the relief she experiences when turning down anxiety-provoking social opportunities. When she chooses to stay home, her suffering initially eases. Then, however, comes the slow burn of despair as she watches time pass while she continues to miss out on all the best things she'd hoped for in her life. Even though she experiences initial relief by avoiding anxiety-provoking social situations, her avoidance is unworkable because it leads to greater suffering over time as her social anxiety continues to grow and the pain of her loneliness grows.

> *Darius is having a panic attack while driving his family to the airport. His twelve-year-old twins are giggling happily in the backseat, as they have been waiting their entire lives for this trip to Disney World. Darius, however, is petrified at the thought of getting on an airplane. His mind tells him over and over about how dangerous flying is and that they will crash if they take today's flight. Yet he knows that these are just thoughts and he is determined to not let his anxiety stop him from taking his family on their dream holiday. He knows that his anxiety may make for a painful journey, but he is determined to board that plane.*
>
> *Even though it was initially uncomfortable, he boldly faced his fear and took the flight. Instead of fighting with his anxiety, he practised gentle acceptance. He gave his family a magical holiday and memories that will last a lifetime.*

Darius made one of the most uncomfortable decisions of his life by getting on that plane. It is very challenging to face a phobia head-on, but he decided it was worth it. Even though it was very emotionally painful at times, his behaviour was workable. It moved him towards his value of being a fun and adventurous dad. Also, it was a step towards reducing his suffering in the future as he wants to take his family on a plane trip each year and he might get offered a promotion at work, which would involve frequent air travel. By taking his first flight in many years,

Darius has taken the first step toward flying with less suffering as he can lessen his phobia over time by regularly facing his fear. In other words, the short-term pain of anxiety during this flight led to many long-term gains in his life.

Choosing your response

Now that you understand who you want to be when distressing moments show up for you, you get to make a choice (keep in mind, the choice is only available to you if you have disengaged your autopilot). The choice is like a fork in the road you are travelling on: one way will take you away from being the person you want to be, the other towards your Best Self.

THE MINDFUL FREAK-OUT

SKILL BUILDING: CHOOSING YOUR BEST SELF RESPONSE

For this exercise, list some common situations that trigger highly distressing moments for you and then identify a Best Self response for each. Here are some examples.

Distressing situation	Desired Best Self response
My doctor asked me to come in to discuss my blood test results.	I would text my best friend for moral support, and keep breathing, and be kind to myself and the people at the doctor's office while waiting to see my doctor.
An argument with my spouse over chores begins to get heated.	I would like to ask for a 5-minute break so I can get more grounded and be less reactive. Then I would like to hear her out and see if we can come up with a compromise. I want to use a calm tone and 'I' statements rather than attack her. Afterwards, I want to let it go for now and focus on connecting deeply with her.
Invited to a party.	I will try to see it as an opportunity to connect with others and say 'yes' to the invitation even though I'll have a strong urge to avoid going.
Driver cut me off in traffic.	I no longer want to be a road-rager. I'll sit with the anger that shows up and work to be more self-compassionate and consider that the other driver is doing the best they can with the life they were randomly born into. I'll resist the urge to get revenge.

Choosing your Best Self response

Now it's your turn.

Distressing situation	Desired Best Self response

THE MINDFUL FREAK-OUT

At times, the Best Self response might be to keep breathing and stay engaged in the present moment activity. For example, you show up at a party and your plus-one turns out to be your social anxiety. Your 'date' is unpleasant, but you know that connecting with people is a huge value of yours. You know that, while it might initially feel good, if you flee the party it will lead to more anxiety next time. And avoiding the party means the loss of opportunities to connect and, perhaps, find a more pleasant dating partner. So you decide to stay put, realizing that the best thing to do right now is nothing (don't leave, don't avoid, don't self-medicate, don't struggle, don't ruminate). Instead, you can keep breathing, focus on the present moment, and make space to feel any difficult emotions that show up.

At other times, your Best Self response in a difficult moment might require taking action that is very much in line with what your threat system recommends. For example, quickly slowing your car when the person in the car in front of you on the highway suddenly slams on their brakes.

The behaviour that is a Best Self action in one situation may be the same behaviour that takes you away from being your Best Self in another situation. For example, avoiding social events that might take you closer to your value of connecting with others would not be acting as your Best Self. On the other hand, avoiding social situations that are hostile or abusive is likely to be both values-consistent and self-compassionate. What is important is having the psychological flexibility to respond adaptively based on your Best Self.

Sometimes, we can get stuck wondering how best to handle a particular distressing situation. For example, let's say that you and your spouse are fighting over which one of you should pick up the kids from school, given that you both have busy schedules. Perhaps it is a fight you have had over and over and it has only served to strain your relationship. Instead, you could offer to sit down together and work as a team to problem-solve the situation without blame. That way you can work on your values of having a close connection to your children and spouse while also ending a cycle of blame, which only increases suffering for both of you.

KEY POINTS

- When feeling highly distressed, often behaviours that lead to immediate relief lead to longer term suffering.

- Rather than reacting based on a strong painful emotion, you can choose to respond based on your Best Self.

- Your Best Self responds based on your core values, with a focus on easing suffering in the long term.

12

COMMITTING TO TAKING ACTION AND NOTICING THE OUTCOME

There is a scene in the movie *Silver Linings Playbook* where the protagonist, Pat, is being baited by his brother, Jake, who is likely playing out a longstanding dysfunctional family dynamic. Pat is newly released from a psychiatric facility where he was being held because he lost control and nearly beat his wife's lover to death. Jake is pushing Pat by describing all the ways his own life is successful compared to Pat's (Jake is getting made partner at his law firm, Pat lost his job; Jake is getting engaged, Pat is separated from his wife; Jake is getting a new house, Pat lost his home). There is a pause as tension seems to heat up and, given Pat's history of explosive anger, his onlooking parents fear he will rage at his brother who is pushing him. Instead, Pat uses the pause to get off autopilot and decide how he wants to handle this potentially volatile situation. Pat then looks his brother in the eyes and with deep sincerity he takes action based on his Best Self, telling his brother, 'I got nothing but love for you, brother,' and then proceeds to give his brother a big hug. Situation defused, suffering minimized, and Pat's values, like his brother, are embraced.

Once you've disengaged your autopilot, made space for the pain that has shown up and with compassion decided who you want to be when times get tough, it is time to act based on your Best Self.

What can help you to take values-based action in a difficult moment?

Practice.

You certainly can choose to wait until you are experiencing a highly distressing moment to begin to act compassionately based on your values. But why wait until then to start living based on what's important to you?

You can prime the pump by committing to taking action today — at least in some small (or big) ways. You completed the values exercises to discover what you want your life to stand for; now let's set some goals that move you in the direction of those values. By doing this, you can begin to build some muscle memory for how you want to act. Then when things get tough you won't have to dig as deep to bring to mind responses that are consistent with you living as your Best Self. The more you use these skills and strategies the more helpful they become and the more likely you are to remember to use them (and use them effectively) when your threat system tries to take over.

The question to ask yourself is: what concrete steps can you take towards living your values today?

Committing to taking action and noticing the outcome

Let's look at some examples:

Sean is painfully socially anxious to the point of not wanting to leave his home. Things have gotten so much worse since the Covid lockdown enabled him to work from home. Now he rarely leaves. His company, however, is now mandating all employees to return to the office beginning in two weeks, and he is distressed to the point of considering quitting his job.

Sean dreams of a life filled with social connection, love and adventure, and would like to start a family. His current reality, however, stands in stark contrast to his deepest wish for how he would like his life to be.

Sean's highly distressing moment will be two weeks from now when he will be asked to get in his car and drive to the office. In his heart of hearts he would like to not only make it to the office on that day, but not let his social anxiety hold him back from his life any longer. He can commit to taking action today that will not only make it easier for him to make it to the office, but also make strides towards his values, such as connecting with others. Today he can begin taking actions, such as:

- calling an old friend on the phone, just to connect
- inviting a co-worker he is friendly with to have coffee
- speaking up on a virtual work meeting (he is usually the quiet one)
- scheduling an appointment with a therapist who can guide him through social anxiety exposure therapy.

THE MINDFUL FREAK-OUT

Raven lives in fear of having a panic attack. When she has one, she feels as if she is going to literally die of fright. Because of this she does not like to leave the few remaining areas in her comfort zone, such as her home and her job. She never knows when a panic attack will strike, and as a result she lives her life in a state of always being on guard.

Yet Raven dreams of travelling the world. She feels like that is what she's been put on this Earth to do, but because of her fear of panic attacks she hasn't left her little town in three years and hasn't driven alone on the highway in ten years. And she can induce a panic attack by just imagining getting on an airplane.

Raven would like to make her life less about her anxiety and more about savouring the big wide world around her. Today she can get started broadening her world. For example, she can:

- make a top five travel adventures list to use as extra motivation to begin facing her anxiety rather than fighting it
- read up on exposure therapy strategies for panic disorder and commit to at least one exposure per day
- hike a new trail
- drive to a nearby town and walk through the town centre
- reach out to her old travel buddy to see if she would be interested in planning a trip
- commit to practising mindful acceptance of smaller daily emotional discomforts.

Committing to taking action and noticing the outcome

Malik has a temper. It doesn't take much to set him off. The bouncer at the club looked at him 'the wrong way' and he saw red and started an argument. The driver in front of him was going below the speed limit – so he sped up and tried to intimidate them into going faster. Then, there was no record of the concert tickets that were supposed to be waiting for him at the box office. His hostile tone and words led to security guards escorting him off the premises. And all of this was just one weekend out of a life filled with rage-fuelled tirades.

On the outside, Malik appears to be a man made of rage. However, what people don't see is the shame he carries with him post-rage. Down deep, Malik is a spiritual person. What is most important to him is his faith, first and foremost. He values compassion, peace and gratitude and how he behaves runs counter to who he wants to be. His regret after impulsively acting on his anger leads him to feeling depressed much of the time. The depression inflames his irritability, which makes him more likely to lash out when triggered. Today he can take the following values-based steps to:

- attend a religious service
- reach out to his spiritual advisor for guidance
- practise kindness and patience with those in his life he cares about
- practise random acts of kindness towards strangers (giving a compliment, slowing down to allow someone to merge in front of him on the highway, leaving an extra big tip along with an encouraging note, going for a walk

and giving a friendly smile to people he passes, and offering his seat to someone else on the train).

SKILL BUILDING:
IDENTIFYING IMMEDIATE VALUES-BASED BEHAVIOURS

Think of some of your core values, which you identified previously. List some ways you can act now on what is important to you, so you can work towards creating a habit of responding to situations in values-based ways. How can you prime your valued-action pump?

-
-
-
-
-
-
-
-
-
-

Barriers to taking values-based action

Why is taking values-based action so difficult in times of emotional intensity and suffering? There are a number of reasons.

1. You are on autopilot

If we cannot get off autopilot then none of the other skills and strategies are available to us at times when we need them the most. You might need to repeatedly consciously disengage your autopilot during difficult moments when your threat system keeps flipping the autopilot switch back on. Review Part 1 for ways to get better at getting off autopilot and getting back in control.

2. You are struggling against the emotional pain – you are unwilling to feel it

It is a natural urge to want to put up a fight when facing the pain that certain emotions bring. Rather than taking value-based action in a distressing situation, we can get distracted by going to war against the emotional pain. Remember, fighting emotional pain, even though it can be a powerful instinct, tends to inflame the suffering instead of soothing it. And while we are battling with ourselves, we are less likely to be acting based on our values. See Chapter 8 for strategies to ease such counterproductive struggle.

3. You are fused with unhelpful content of the mind

'I can't do this!'

'This anxiety will kill me!'

'I need to be the best or else!'

Our minds are chatterboxes and at times they tell us some very dark and distressing things. You and I and everyone are all in the same boat with this. There is no escaping having a noisy and often unhelpful mind. If you buy what your mind is selling, however, you are more likely to engage in emotion-driven behaviour. However, you can learn to get some distance between yourself and unhelpful thoughts. Defusing from these thoughts can give you the space and opportunity to have choice in your response to highly distressing moments. See Chapter 9 for strategies to help you defuse from unhelpful thoughts.

4. You haven't clarified your values

Without defining who you want to be and what you want to stand for during your time on this planet, you are at the whim of automatic reactions when things get intense. By defining what you want your life to stand for, you then have a built-in guide for how to respond to life's curveballs. See p. 178 for ways to identify your core values.

5. You are not completely sold on the idea of behaving differently in your triggering situations

All things being equal, behaviour doesn't change. Change is often difficult, especially when that change involves turning and facing distressing thoughts and painful feelings.

So what's in it for you to make a change in how you respond to intense emotions? Look back to the exercise 'Choosing your Best Self response on p. 168. Now ask yourself, what's in it for you to choose this response over your threat-based automatic reaction?

Here are some examples:

Situation	Past response	Costs of my typical response	Chosen Best Self response	Potential pay-offs for Best Self response
My doctor asked me to come in to discuss my blood test results.	I panicked alone in my room, hyperventilating in a foetal position on the bed. When I went to the doctor's office, I snapped at the receptionist because the doctor was not on time.	I felt terribly alone and miserable. I felt bad about snapping at the receptionist; it was not her fault.	I would text my best friend for moral support, and keep breathing, and be kind to myself and the people at the doctor's office while waiting to see my doctor.	It could bring me and my friend closer together. It would be nice having someone supportive to talk to. I might feel less miserable if I am kind to myself and other people.
An argument with my spouse over chores begins to get heated.	I start to yell, which shuts him down. I say really mean things to him which I later regret. Our relationship seems worse for a week or two after the argument.	I get down on myself for the mean things I said. My spouse is my best friend and life is more painful when we are not getting along.	I would like to ask for a 5-minute break so I can get more grounded and be less reactive. Then I would like to hear him out and see if we can come up with a compromise. I want to use a calm tone and use 'I' statements rather than attack him. Afterwards, I want to let it go for now and focus on connecting deeply with him.	We may argue less often. Improve our relationship. And perhaps work out a way to address chores that we both feel good about. Also, I'll feel less guilty about my behaviour afterwards.

THE MINDFUL FREAK-OUT

Invited to a party.	Most of the time I automatically come up with an excuse about why I can't make it.	I feel lonelier and more depressed.	I will try to see it as an opportunity to connect with others and say 'yes' to the invitation even though I'll have a strong urge to avoid going.	I might make some more friends and deepen existing friendships. Perhaps I'll find a romantic partner.
Driver cut me off in traffic.	I drove close behind them and continued to honk the horn. Then I pulled alongside, rolled down my window and yelled at her!	I felt angry for the next few days. My family saw me acting horribly and don't want to ride with me when I am driving.	I no longer want to be a road rager. I'll sit with the anger that shows up and work to be more self-compassionate and consider that the other driver is doing the best they can with the life they were randomly born into. I'll resist the urge to get revenge.	I won't feel like an out-of-control angry dude. I'll be able to let it go easier. It may help my blood pressure. I won't risk getting into a physical fight.

Now think of some of your own responses:

Situation	Past response	Costs of my typical response	Chosen Best Self response	Potential pay-offs for Best Self response

When you compare the pay-offs of your Best Self response to the costs of your typical reaction, which strategy moves you closer to the life you want to live?

6. There is another practical barrier in the way
Let's say you have a goal of responding to distressing interpersonal situations with assertiveness in the service of your value of peace or connection — but you don't have the skills yet. That is a barrier to you responding how you would like to respond. Or perhaps you value adventure and would like to face your fear of the unknown and travel internationally for the first time, but cannot currently afford it. That is a barrier to your desired adventure and to facing your fear of the unknown.

Overcoming your barriers

What barriers stand between you and values-based action in the face of highly distressing moments? Give some thought to what they are and how you might be able to handle those barriers. Is there a problem that needs to be solved or a decision that needs to be made? Or is it a matter of deciding which ACT and CFT strategies will be most useful and practising them ahead of time? For example:

Committing to taking action and noticing the outcome

Distressing situation	Desired Best Self response	Barriers that might be present	How I can handle the barriers
My doctor asked me to come in to discuss my blood test results.	I would text my best friend for moral support, and keep breathing, and be kind to myself and the people at the doctor's office while waiting to see my doctor.	My friend might not be available and I might forget to use a centring breath and practise kindness.	I can choose some other people to call if my best friend is not available. I can make a note in my phone to remind myself of my valued strategies when stressful situations like this arise.
Disagreement with my spouse over chores.	I would like to ask for a 5-minute break so I can get more grounded and be less reactive. Then I would like to hear her out and see if we can come up with a compromise. I want to use a calm tone and use 'I' statements rather than attack her. Afterwards, I want to let it go for now and focus on connecting deeply with her.	Feelings of anger, judgmental thoughts, and a powerful urge to get my way makes it difficult to get off autopilot.	Accept the feelings and remember that they are not my fault and I don't have to let them run my life. Use defusion imagery, like leaves on a stream, to unhook from the thoughts and urges. I can take a break if I need to so I can remind myself of what is truly important in my life.
Invited to a party.	I will try to see it as an opportunity to connect with others and say 'yes' to the invitation even though I'll have a strong urge to avoid going.	I might automatically turn down the invitation.	I'll make a habit of saying, 'That sounds like fun, I'll check my schedule and get back to you.' Later, I can use compassion skills to bolster my courage to say 'yes'.

THE MINDFUL FREAK-OUT

| Driver cut me off in traffic. | I no longer want to be a road rager. I'll sit with the anger that shows up and work to be more self-compassionate and consider that the other driver is doing the best they can with the life they were randomly born into. I'll resist the urge to get revenge. | In the heat of the moment, I might forget to act based on my Best Self. | I can begin to practise mindfulness and compassionate actions towards others. I can put a reminder on the dashboard of my car in big, bold letters. |

Now think about some of your own barriers and write down how you might be able to handle them.

Distressing situation	Desired Best Self response	Barriers that might be present	How I can handle the barriers

7. You are caught in the all-or-nothing perfectionism trap
Sometimes our minds make perfectionistic rules for us such as:

- 'I need to do this perfectly or not at all!'
- 'If I'm unable to do it 100 percent of the time then I've failed!'
- 'A slip up means I can't do it — so I should just give up!'

The problem is, we *are* imperfect and we *will* slip up. So these perfectionistic rules are unworkable. Think *progress — not perfection* — as the goal to strive for. Try to learn from freak-out moments that don't go well — and return to self-compassion *unconditionally*.

Noticing the outcome

Now that you have begun to respond to challenging moments from a Best Self perspective rather than impulsively reacting based on emotion, the key question is not 'Is this harder than acting on impulse?'. Sometimes it will be and other times not. Moving towards what's important to you, especially in the presence of painful emotions, can be difficult, but so are many profoundly important life goals such as having children, going to school, attending a job interview or maintaining a long-term relationship. In a sense, it would be *easier* to just not go after these things.

The key question is whether responding based on your Best Self is moving your life in a valued direction while addressing your suffering over time. ACT therapist Tobias Lundgren uses the analogy of a dartboard.[1] The centre of the dartboard, the bullseye, indicates that you believe you are choosing actions that are completely consistent with your values. If you hit the ring around the bullseye, you are getting very close! The further away from the bullseye, the further away you are from choosing actions that are consistent with what you want your life to stand for.

During your most recent highly distressing moment, how close did you come to a bullseye? What can you do to get closer next time?

Noticing what happens after taking action helps maximize your growth

New and more adaptive learning can come from facing a difficult situation. This new learning can further ease your suffering over time. If you are agoraphobic and fear leaving a narrow comfort zone like your home, it is wonderful when you choose to move out into the broader world. Facing limiting fears like this is highly self-compassionate. It means you are willing to do something difficult now (facing your fear) so that your life has less suffering in the future.

According to Dr Michelle Craske's inhibitory learning research, taking the time to notice the outcome after taking action offers the potential for extra growth as you deepen your safety learning.[2] In other words, it can help you to be less afraid in the future if after each time you face a fear you take a moment to consider:

1. 'Did the worst-case scenario that my mind was worried about actually happen?'
2. 'Even if it was uncomfortable, was I able to tolerate the experience?'

By taking time to notice 'It wasn't as bad as I thought' and 'I didn't like how it felt but I could tolerate it', you are a step closer towards decreasing the fear of that situation. This translates into less suffering in the future.

In the next chapter, we will discuss more about how you can turn highly distressing moments into growth opportunities. Then we will look at some common sources of freak-outs and which behaviours can help lead to more personal growth.

KEY POINTS

- Intentionally practising values-based behaviours during non-freak-out times can prepare you for taking values-based action during highly distressing moments.

- There are often barriers to values-based behaviours in difficult moments. By anticipating your barriers, you can practise skills ahead of time to overcome those barriers.

13

NAVIGATING COMMON FREAK-OUTS

Eliza is freaking out! She texted her boyfriend an hour ago – and still no response! She feels very worried that something is wrong, that either he has been in an accident or perhaps he is breaking up with her. After centring herself and engaging her compassionate mind to turn towards her suffering she notices that she feels a strong urge to text over and over until he responds. Instead of giving in to this urge she decides to call a friend to chat and perhaps make dinner plans (she later learns he had no phone reception while on a work assignment).

In this chapter we will review helpful responses to common freak-outs. Please note, these are general suggestions based on ACT, CFT, and also research on exposure therapy. They are meant to be flexibly applied. This means that what is workable for you one day in a particular context may be unhelpful for you on a different day in a different context.

For example, you might find that in some contexts walking away during a conflict is a workable solution (someone bumps into you while walking and you experience rage that threatens to push you into a physical altercation). In another context, standing your ground is a more workable solution than walking away (you are a teacher and your student blatantly cheated on their exam).

There will be some moments when you realize that your autopilot feels overpowering. In these moments the action you choose to take might be to re-cycle through the steps of compassionate awareness and compassionate acceptance. Things might be so hot that you need more time to cool off and get centred. If, in the heat of the moment, you believe you won't be able to stop yourself from behaving aggressively, then a prolonged break can be values-consistent and address your suffering over the long term (you may suffer more if you break up with your partner on impulse during a difficult moment or punch your neighbour whose dog just pooped on your lawn).

Using difficult moments as an AFGO

Underneath highly distressing moments is a hidden opportunity for growth. When you face a fear, for example, you have the opportunity to learn that you can tolerate it and that catastrophe is unlikely to occur. When you face a distressing feeling with compassionate willingness, you can likewise learn that you can bear the weight — and even notice that with greater compassion and willingness you are likely to suffer much less. This is a profound life lesson to experience and learn from. You can even learn that in the face of discomfort, you can be kind to yourself and others, and move forward with valued goals despite the discomfort. That's growth.

AFGO is an acronym that stands for Another Freaking Growth Opportunity. Some use the word 'Freeing' instead of 'Freaking' while others use a much less polite word. This captures the spirit of the challenging situation: 'This moment is difficult, but I will choose to make the best of it and try to take away something useful from it.'

My biggest fear for much of my younger life was flying. Well, to be specific the fear was less about flying and more about suddenly and dramatically not flying — falling from 30,000 feet! Turbulence equalled terror for me. The biggest part of my recovery from this fear was learning to see turbulence as an opportunity to face my biggest fear, so I could be free to fly where and when I wanted. When the captain would announce it would be a bumpy flight, I would sigh and tell myself, 'Okay, let's do this'. It became an opportunity to show myself that I could survive a bumpy flight.

Training your threat system

Your threat system is like a fiercely loyal, ever-vigilant guard dog. When it thinks there is a threat, it will howl and activate your fight-or-flight response to flood you with adrenaline so that you can take quick action to protect yourself. The problem is that our threat system does not reside in the smart part of our brain. It resides in a much more primitive part of our brain (called the limbic system), where it quite often misperceives threats. Have you ever had the experience of being on a hike, seeing a curvy stick on the ground in front of you and before you register it as a stick, your inner guard dog howls, '*Snake!*'? Have you ever been a passenger in a car with a driver you were not comfortable with, and on reflex used your leg to push the imaginary brake pedal in front of you? Or how about when watching a horror movie and your body floods you with energy to prepare you to fight off the monster that only exists on the screen in front of you? Like I said, the threat system is not in the smart part of the brain!

That said, it still learns — all the time. If you are terrified of public speaking and are asked to give a speech at your best friend's wedding, the action you take will either teach your threat system that public speaking is reasonably safe (if you follow through with giving the speech) or it will continue to teach your threat system that public speaking is dangerous (if you choose to avoid giving the speech). It will learn something either way. The question is, what do you want it to learn by your behaviour?

Your threat system can learn many useful things. However, it will always remain in the more primitive part of your brain. It will always be glitchy and say and do silly things at times. Therefore, you don't have to pressure yourself to make the guard dog perfect before you pursue what you want (and what it fears) such as love, career, adventure and other important values. You can take steps now to pursue what is important to you, glitchy friend in tow, while you teach it a few helpful things along the way.

Now let's explore some common freak-outs and growth-oriented actions you could choose to take.

The freak-out: Panic attacks

Panic attacks are quick surges of intense fear that reach a peak within minutes and bring with them a range of physical symptoms such as increased heart rate, shaking, sweating, shortness of breath and so on. They can be profoundly distressing experiences that leave some people so shaken up that they live in fear of having more attacks. During a panic attack the person might get hooked by thoughts such as, 'I'm losing control, I'm going crazy' or even, 'I'm going to die!' These can be truly terrifying experiences.

When someone has a panic attack, they are experiencing a powerful full-body and mind reaction to a perceived (or misperceived) threat. For some, this bodily reaction is experienced in the context of entertainment — it feels terrifyingly thrilling. Think of the roller-coaster riders, bungee jumpers and sky divers gleefully screaming as they fall, bounce and plummet. For others, a panic attack means they are face to face with something they are very afraid of (turbulence on a plane, a spider crawling on their arm, or giving a presentation in front of a room full of people). They are focused on the scary thing and less concerned about their intense bodily reaction (the panic attack).

And then there are those who are intensely afraid of the panic attack itself. While some may feel panicked by turbulence on an airplane out of fear that the plane might fall, others are so afraid of the panic attack itself that they panic in trying to fight off the panic. For them, their fear is of the fear itself, because they believe panic attacks are dangerous to their physical or mental health.

But while panic attacks can feel scary, they are in fact very safe to experience. Those bungee jumpers and roller-coaster riders are having the physical equivalent of a panic attack. Can you imagine how tragic the thrill rides at Disneyland would be if our body's fight-or-flight response was actually as dangerous as it sometimes feels?

Intense fight-or-flight responses are how we have always survived in a world filled with danger. This is our body's ingenious way to quickly fill us with the energy, strength and focus needed to overcome a threat. Mother nature would have created a very shoddy safety device (our nervous systems) if, when we were fighting or fleeing from a threat, we just keeled over and died because of the adrenaline surge.

When autopilot takes control

When you feel a panic attack coming, your threat system will try to take over. If it succeeds, it could drive you to avoid whatever is triggering the anxiety *and* it will likely push you into a battle against your fear, leading you to struggle against your own body to try to get rid of the anxiety. However, the harder you fight anxiety or a full-blown panic attack, the more intense they can get — and the more suffering they bring. Part of the problem is that when you tense up because you are struggling with anxiety, you dysregulate your breathing, which can further activate your sympathetic nervous system, dumping even more anxiety onto anxiety.[1]

People who fear panic attacks might use other avoidant strategies when they fear they will have a panic attack. For example, they might make sure to always have a full water bottle with them when they leave home to try to ward off anxiety. They might try to distract themselves or seek reassurance by phoning a 'safe person'. In addition to such external safety behaviours, people with panic disorder engage in internal safety behaviours such as struggling with their anxiety, over-monitoring their body sensations ('What's my heart doing? How am I feeling? Is an attack coming?') and desperately trying to force themselves to relax.

Avoidance behaviours often might ease people's suffering — in the short term (for example, feeling more relaxed after cancelling social plans out of fear of having a panic attack and being away from home).

Although avoiding a triggering place or situation may work well for temporarily relieving anxiety, it further trains the threat system to fear such experiences *and* it keeps people away from valued life goals. Such avoidance can teach a person's threat system to be so wary of panic attacks that they develop full-on agoraphobia, where people can be deathly afraid of stepping outside of their shrinking comfort zone. I have a relative who has barely left her home in five years, and there are people around the world who have felt trapped in their narrow comfort zones for decades.

Helpful action
Choosing to take helpful action in the face of a panic attack may mean seeing the panic attack as an exposure therapy opportunity. Exposure therapy for a fear of panic attacks involves facing internal triggers, which are typically those bodily sensations people associate with a panic attack (elevated heart rate, dizziness, lightheadedness, and so on) they have been trying to avoid feeling. Facing external triggers is also an important part of exposure therapy for panic fears. The external triggers most often are those places and situations associated with panic attacks. These are often places where 'escape' feels more difficult like stadiums, airplanes or the back of a large store.

You can choose to methodically face the feared places and situations, starting with something relatively less triggering, and work your way on up to bigger challenges. Alternatively, instead of starting with something easier, you can plan values-based exposures. For example, if you can plan a trip to visit a dear friend who is ill, you are still facing a range of fears, but it is in the service of something directly meaningful to you.

In addition to seeking out exposure challenges, exposure therapy also involves making the best of unexpected triggers or panic attacks that seem to randomly show up. Rather than seeing an out-of-the-blue panic attack as your enemy to be struggled with, you can choose to see it as an opportunity to practise your skills and provide your threat system with a teachable moment — showing it that although panic attacks are uncomfortable, they are time-limited, are not deadly, and are relatively tolerable when met with acceptance, non-struggle, non-judgment, defusion and compassion. Acceptance does not mean liking or wanting a panic attack; it simply means making space for whatever the reality of the moment is without inflaming your suffering through struggle.

The freak-out: Being in the social spotlight

Social anxiety, while uncomfortable, is a normal part of human life. In fact, social situations, like public speaking, are among the most common sources of anxiety. Why would social situations be so anxiety provoking for so many people? It is because social situations used to be far riskier than they are today.

Remember, for the vast majority of time humans have been on this planet we were hunters and gatherers banded together in small nomadic tribes living in a dangerous and resource-deprived world. If one of our distant ancestors was out hunting and gathering and found a large berry bush, they would have wanted to collect that precious nutrition to bring back to their small tribe. If a stranger from another tribe happened upon them, also hungry due to a scarcity of food, that situation could have easily turned into a 'kill or be killed' moment. Being wary of outsiders would have been adaptive.

However, even within their own tribes, our ancestors would have wanted to be careful not to behave in a way to upset the tribe. Displeasing the tribe could lead to banishment — and guess how long our prehistoric ancestors could survive without the mutual protection of other people? Not long! So it would have been adaptive to have enough social concern (i.e. social anxiety) to motivate our ancestors to not disrespect the tribe and risk being expelled. Likewise, having social concerns when picking a mate would have made sense. These were small tribes and there would have been competition for a very limited number of possible mates. Getting rejected would have greatly diminished potential mating opportunities. They certainly weren't going to fire up a dating app and message the attractive person in the neighbouring tribe.

Social anxiety has always been an adaptive part of human life and most of us can relate to it today. Most of us feel uncomfortable in certain social contexts, at least some of the time to some degree. For others, it can become downright phobic and lead to either significant social avoidance or attending feared social situations with great discomfort.

When autopilot takes control

When social anxiety takes over and puts you on autopilot, it will try to get you to avoid those social situations that *it* misperceives to be threatening. This can lead people to hold off on dating, education or career, making friends or other valued activities. They get fused with thoughts such as:

- 'I will be humiliated.'
- 'I can't tolerate rejection.'
- 'I'm too weird, boring or awkward.'

THE MINDFUL FREAK-OUT

People can come to mistakenly believe that if they hold off facing uncomfortable situations for now, one day they will feel ready to go after their social goals. However, it typically doesn't work that way. The more you avoid uncomfortable social situations the more ingrained the fears become.

You might choose to face the fears, but use other avoidant behaviours such as:

- **drinking alcohol** *before* **a social event**
- **helping out in the kitchen to avoid making small talk at a party**
- **speaking quickly to rush through a presentation**
- **trying to be socially perfect**
- **wearing extra make-up to cover up blushing.**

As seductive as avoidance can feel in the face of social discomfort, it comes at a high cost. The more you avoid uncomfortable social situations the scarier they become and the more you miss out on valued social goals.

Helpful action
Autopilot will try to steer you away from social situations that it misperceives to be a threat. The best way to overcome a social fear is to face it. That means taking steps towards your social goals while allowing for your threat emotions to sound off in the background. If you notice that your anxiety implores you to act perfectly, allow yourself to be yourself — flaws and all.

Over time, you might notice these situations feel less and less threatening and, meanwhile, you have taken steps towards the life you desire. This can only happen if you treat uncomfortable social situations as an AFGO.

The middle-of-the-night freak-out: Insomnia distress

> It's three o'clock in the morning and Caroline is at her wit's end! She has been tossing and turning for hours and she still can't fall asleep. She's tried everything she can think of: counting sheep, listening to peaceful music, reading a book and so much more, but here she is, more wide awake than before! She begins to panic. 'What if I don't sleep at all! How will I be able to function at work? If I don't sleep I won't be able to make it through the day!' She gets out of bed and begins to pace, hoping she can wear herself out. Now she's even more wide awake! 'I can't take this!' she frets. She calls her sister, who is sound asleep, 'I need to sleep! What can I do?' Her sister is concerned, but also very annoyed as she has to get up in a few hours herself. Her sister gives out advice, which Caroline swats away. 'I tried that!' she snaps, upsetting her sister, who hangs up. Caroline stares helplessly at the clock, 'I can't take this – I need to sleep right now!'

I have a riddle for you: *The harder you chase me the further away I get. The more you struggle to tame me, the wilder I get. What am I?*

The answer is sleep.

There are few things I see in my psychology private practice that are as distressing for people as persistent insomnia. Being sleep deprived can feel physically and mentally very unpleasant, so it makes sense that people would feel a powerful urge to fight off insomnia. They toss and turn and stare at their clocks in frustration. They try strategy after strategy to force their insomnia to leave and never return. So often, however, these attempts to control their insomnia inflame it. As the poor sleep spreads into multiple nights, the ferocity with which they try to control their sleep grows with each restless night.

I can recall as a college student I went through a prolonged period of struggling with my sleep. I tried through sheer grit and determination to force myself to sleep — to no avail. I tossed and turned, I paced, I counted thousands of imaginary sheep, I wracked my brain nightly trying to remember the 'secret' to sleep that I thought I must have known at one time.

What young-me did not realize was that we don't control our sleep. Our bodies are responsible for sleep, not us. We can set the stage by practising good sleep hygiene such as having our bedrooms dark and cool, and minimizing substances like caffeine, which makes sleep more difficult. But, like me in college, many people with persistent insomnia treat sleeplessness like a battle against an unseen enemy.

When autopilot takes control
When autopilot takes over, trying to protect you from the 'threat' of insomnia, it means getting hooked by thoughts such as:

- 'If I don't sleep I will have an awful day!'
- 'I must get enough sleep or else something terrible will happen!'

- 'Being sleep deprived is intolerable!'
- 'I may never get a good night's sleep again!'

Then comes the struggle — tossing and turning, tense and desperate. Clock watching and mental calculations of how much sleep you will get if you only fell asleep *now* — only to see the minutes and hours tick away. People get trapped in a paradox. The more they *must* sleep the more wide awake they become. The harder they fight with their insomnia, the more stress hormones course through their veins, creating increased wakefulness.

Remember: sleep is not something you do. It is something your body does when you get out of its way.

Helpful action

We want to associate sleep (or lack of sleep) with safety rather than threat. That way, you are less likely to have a fight-or-flight reaction in response to those times when insomnia decides to pay a visit. When we behave as if it is a threat, it is more likely to become a chronic source of suffering. People with insomnia often try to take control of their sleep, but by trying to control it they run the risk of turning insomnia into an enemy, thus bringing on more wakefulness. Instead of meeting insomnia with struggle, you can learn to meet it with compassionate acceptance, as it is common for insomnia to show up periodically.

Sleep specialist Dr Guy Meadows recommends that you do nothing to try to control sleep.[2] He warns that it is easy to turn useful strategies into unhelpful control strategies. So while watching caffeine and nicotine intake, easing up on technology before bed, and avoiding excessive napping can be helpful, using these strategies as a way to ensure there will be no insomnia (that is, to try to control it) can backfire. Instead, you can take some steps to make your environment and body more sleep-friendly and then get out of the way.

Instead of focusing on struggling with or controlling your insomnia, Dr Meadows recommends taking a mindful approach (using strategies similar to those in this book) to make space for whatever emotions or sensations show up, without bracing against them or judging them. Rather than checking the clock and struggling when you cannot sleep, you can shift your focus to what you can see behind your closed eyelids, the swirling shapes and colours. You can notice sounds in the room and further away. You can notice the temperature in the room, the softness of the mattress, the fluffiness of your pillow, and the feel of your pyjamas on your body. You can also notice the sensations you experience inside your body and watch them as they shift and fluctuate. You can notice what it feels like to soften into the restorative embrace of gentle rest.

Another way to conceptualize this is through the CFT Three-System Model of Emotion Regulation (see p. 89). From a CFT perspective, you can meet your insomnia with your threat system, which dumps activating cortisol into your system, making sleep more elusive. You can meet your insomnia with the drive system, coming at it with tenacity and problem-solving, with a keen determination to outsmart your 'opponent' and seize the prize of sleep. The problem is that the effort to defeat your insomnia is likely to crank up the volume on your nervous system, which pushes sleep further from your grasp. Or you can meet your insomnia with the more kind and gentle compassion system (see p. 100 for strategies). This can lead to a release of oxytocin, which is more likely to bring soothing to your nervous system, making conditions for sleep more favourable.[3]

In addition, you can choose to use the day after a night of insomnia as another AFGO. You may be tempted to struggle with what you feel the next day. Instead, unhook from the catastrophic story your mind is telling you about the intolerability of the moment. Then, focus mindfully on your senses and your breath. Let go of the struggle with your sleepy self. Sit softly with what you actually feel and allow the 'I can't stand this' thoughts to come and go. If you hook onto the unhelpful thoughts, acknowledge the thought without judgment ('There is thought') and come back to your body as it is.

What do you notice?

Likely you are feeling sleepy, but you may also notice that, underneath the struggle, sleep deprivation can feel mellow and relaxing. Maybe not what you would like if you have a fast-paced day planned, but it's likely that settling into the mellow and relaxing feelings is more desirable than the suffering that comes with struggle. Can you allow for a little of those mellow and relaxing sensations even as you go through your busy day? Who says you have to struggle and suffer because you are tired?

Then, from a perspective of compassion, can you bring some extra nurturing to yourself on this day of feeling tired? Can you treat yourself to one of your favourite lunches? What else would feel nurturing? Perhaps calling a cherished friend or family member to catch up? Also from a compassionate perspective, could you care enough about yourself to not inadvertently perpetuate insomnia by loading up with caffeine and taking a huge nap during the day?

At the end of the day, take notice that your day was less awful than the catastrophic nightmare your mind imagined it would be. You might find it actually was an okay day, which makes insomnia less intimidating so your mind may be less freaked out about the possibility of future nights with poor sleep. When you are less concerned about sleep, you're more likely to sleep.

While it is normal to go through periods of insomnia, chronic insomnia may require some outside help. The most helpful action could be to make an appointment to see your doctor. There are medical conditions, like sleep apnea, that can make sleep much more difficult. Likewise, many common medications and supplements can create sleep problems, which your doctor can help identify and offer advice on.

If your doctor rules out a physical cause to the persistent insomnia, your next best step might be to consult a mental health provider who specializes in insomnia treatment. The good news is that non-medical treatment for insomnia can be extremely effective, such as Cognitive Behavioural Therapy for insomnia (CBT-I).[4] This has been shown to be the gold standard treatment for primary insomnia (insomnia not related to another condition). ACT for insomnia (ACT-I) has a growing research base showing that it is also helpful.[5]

The freak-out at 30,000 feet: Turbulence on your flight

I have had my freak-outs in life just like we all have. However, nothing has created such panic and terror for me as a turbulent flight used to. In my childhood, though, I considered turbulence to be soothing. It would rock me to sleep. However, at age nineteen I took a flight that changed how my brain perceived turbulence. It no longer represented soothing. In my mind it began to represent the terror of crashing.

Ultimately, for most people the fear of flying in a plane is not really about crashing and dying. Most frightened flyers intellectually know that flying is the safest form of travel. The challenge is not one of actual safety; it is about tolerating the *fear* of crashing. Even though the logical part of one's brain may know they are safe, the more primitive part can believe otherwise and activates intense levels of fight-or-flight.

When autopilot takes control
As we've discussed, your threat system tries to take over whenever it feels you are in danger. For many people, flying *feels* dangerous. It's not, but it can feel that way, especially during heavy turbulence when your giant multi-tonne metal flying bus feels like it is being thrown around wildly in the sky.

If you are afraid of flying, even the thought of flying leads your threat system to go to work. First, it tries to convince you to avoid making travel plans or to cancel at the last minute because it doesn't 'feel right'. The relief you get from avoiding airplane travel further trains your threat system to see flying as dangerous and something to avoid. The longer the avoidance goes on, the more flying gets built up as a threat.

As with other sources of anxiety, using safety behaviours while flying can also build up the threat. This was certainly the case for me, who seldom avoided flights, but leaned on safety behaviours to try to avoid the feelings of fear and uncertainty that were my travelling companions. Paradoxically, these made the trips feel even more threatening. Examples of safety behaviours on flights include:

- **tightly gripping the armrests (white knuckle flying)**
- **staring at a screen or magazine to try to forget you're on a plane**
- **compulsively reminding yourself that flying is safe**

THE MINDFUL FREAK-OUT

- analyzing every bump on the flight to determine whether the flight is still safe.

The result of the avoidance and safety behaviours is that opportunities are missed by avoiding flying, and the suffering before and during flights is exacerbated.

Helpful action

If you are a freak-out flier, like I used to be, you likely have tried the avoidance and/or safety behaviour strategy that was encouraged by your threat system. And likely, it hasn't helped you fly more comfortably in the long run. If you wish to suffer less on planes I encourage you to choose a different response to the anxiety that soars along with your flight.

Instead of aiming for a quick fix by using avoidance strategies you can choose to take more helpful action. That might mean making an appointment with a phobia specialist to design an exposure plan. Such a plan might involve looking at images of flying, watching videos and perhaps taking some virtual reality flights. Ultimately, it will mean getting on an airplane. While doing these exposures, ACT encourages shifting your focus from how to fly comfortably to flying for a values-based reason (for example, flying to visit cherished family or friends, or perhaps planning an adventure is meaningful to you).

CFT recommends being self-compassionate when it comes to the fear you feel. Right now, your body has been conditioned to activate the fight-or-flight response around flying. Rather than going to war with anxiety and uncertainty, use the flight as an AFGO. Choose to unclench your muscles, come back to the present moment, and then focus on valued activities such as chatting with a loved one or playing a card game with your child. When the plane hits turbulence and you notice that struggle is occurring, cycle back through compassionate awareness and acceptance skills and then shift back towards the valued activity.

The freak-out: Death and existential panic

We humans typically do not like uncertainty. And there is no greater uncertainty than the big existential uncertainties that surround human life and death:

- What happens when we die?
- Is there a heaven and, if so, will I go there?
- What will it be like to be in heaven for eternity? Will it get boring? Will there be good Wi-Fi reception? How will I spend my time?
- What if there is non-existence — what will that be like?
- What will my death be like — will I suffer?
- What is my purpose on Earth?
- Will I go to hell if I do or don't do this or that? What would that be like?
- If the universe has countless planets with countless species, does my little life here on this planet matter?
- If I'm going to die someday, does anything matter?

While these are the types of questions people contemplate in the course of their life, for some there is an urgency behind it. They must know with certainty the right answer to these big existential questions. For them, not having this certainty can trigger panic — they feel they need to know, right now!

For many people around the world, religion becomes a comforting refuge from existential dread. However, many people have difficulty embracing a 'faith'. Faith implies not knowing for sure. Because of this, for the existentially anxious 'faith' offers little to no comfort. They don't want faith, they want certainty. Which, of course, is impossible.

When autopilot takes control
Existential panic can lead to autopilot taking over, sending the existentially anxious person on a desperate quest for certainty. People attempt to come up with the exact answers to life's big existential questions. This is not done in the slow, methodical, contemplative way philosophers have been doing since the dawn of philosophy. Existential panic is about running away as fast as possible from the experience of uncertainty and towards the impossible goal of absolute certainty.

In the midst of an existential panic people might go down the endless loop of researching on the internet, hoping to find that one piece of information that brings with it freedom from uncertainty. The more time spent trying to get certainty, however, the more uncertain they feel as their uncertainty tolerance muscles continue to atrophy. They may consult priests, rabbis and imams. They may seek out a wide range of gurus, TV therapists and shamans. They might meditate, pray or try out any number of rituals or practices that promise to be the thing that finally relieves them of this cosmic uncertainty Yet, their uncertainty and panic only grows.

Helpful action

If you are someone who experiences existential panic, taking helpful or Best Self action means learning to live with 'faith'. That does not mean you must embrace a spiritual tradition (though you can if you'd like). What it means is learning to turn towards the feelings of uncertainty when they show up — leaning into them rather than struggling against them. It means changing your relationship with existential uncertainty from something you do battle with to something you begin to co-exist with without figuring 'it' out. It means giving up the fantasy of absolute certainty. Then, in the face of the uncertainty, choosing to move towards a life that is filled with valued goals (even as you embrace the uncertainty of whether they are the 'right' goals).

In doing this you build your existential uncertainty-tolerance muscles while moving towards a life you value.

The rage freak-out: Handling your inner Hulk

One of my inspirations for writing this book was the increasing incidence of people raging on airplanes and in stores, sometimes because they didn't want to wear a mask for Covid prevention, or because they wanted someone else to wear a mask, and sometimes just because of the stress of life during the global pandemic.

What we saw on the news and viral videos was presented as a 'bad' person behaving badly. However, some expressed deep remorse and begged people not to judge them based on their worst moment. When watching the videos one thing seems clear: in many cases these were people who were hijacked by their rage, which drove their behaviours in a way that led to public condemnation and, for some, high fines or imprisonment. I think everyone can agree that these were certainly not their best moments.

In places where cameras are not rolling, there are fed-up parents who scream at their children — only to feel ashamed of their behaviour when the rage lets go of them. There are stressed-out teens who unload on a friend during a bad moment, to then be excluded from that friendship group. There are people in loving relationships who get into shouting matches over who left the cap off the toothpaste, only to later wonder why they got so mad over something so trivial.

Like everyone, you might sometimes get taken over by anger and respond in a values-inconsistent way with someone you care about. You might later regret your words or actions, apologize, and wonder how you could have behaved in such a way. I recall hearing the story of the Dalai Lama, a person who has spent most of his life practising deep meditative and compassionate practices, who got angry when fixing a watch because he dropped a screw into the mechanism. In a fit of rage he picked up a hammer and destroyed the precious watch. If it can happen to him, it can happen to any one of us.

The ability to get very angry (like all emotions) is built into us as a way to help us survive and thrive. If we or someone we love is being attacked or oppressed, anger shows up to shut down fear and energize and encourage us to stand up for what and who is important to us. When a military wants to send their young soldiers to war (a truly horrifying experience) they crank up the anger towards the 'enemy' to create animosity, which emboldens these young people to risk their lives while trying to take the lives of others.

However, as with anxiety, anger can flare up intensely for reasons much more trivial than survival. Compassion Focused Therapy reminds us that we were designed this way. It is not our fault — and we are not bad because of having a feeling that was built into us. However, it is our responsibility to try to be aware of our anger and to direct ourselves in a helpful way when our inner Hulk wakes up and wants to smash things.

When autopilot takes control
When anger takes over, it can very quickly escalate a tense situation and direct verbal or physical aggression towards strangers, perceived 'others', loved ones or even ourselves. This is sparked by a perceived injustice ('They looked at me the wrong way!') and inflamed by the instinct to expel the painful feelings of anger. There is a childhood game you may remember called Hot Potato. In this game children sit in a circle and when tossed a ball, they pretend it is so painfully hot that they quickly foist it upon someone else in the group.

Anger can be like that. We often try to run from the intensity of the emotional discomfort by quickly and automatically struggling with it or hurling it aggressively at someone else. We feel bad so we lash out. In the moment, this can release some of the emotional steam that has built up. However, it often leaves us feeling worse in the long run — and it has the potential to damage relationships, threaten our jobs, our self-image, and in some cases results in imprisonment.

Hardly worth the brief relief of releasing the emotional steam.

Helpful action
As difficult as it may be at times, we can get better at getting off autopilot and, instead of striking out in anger (physically or verbally), choose a more values-consistent response. Imagine you were on a game show called 'Make Me Angry' where you were going to be repeatedly insulted

THE MINDFUL FREAK-OUT

with the goal of trying to goad you into an angry outburst. In this imaginary game show, if you can make it past 10 minutes without losing your cool you would win a $20 million cash prize. It is a safe bet that most people, even those with a wild temper, would be able to win that prize.

Now, if in the heat of the moment you are having difficulty staying off autopilot and are at risk of exacerbating a situation with an impulsive angry gesture, sometimes the wisest of actions is to physically remove yourself from the situation if possible. Walk away and re-centre yourself. Sure, this can be difficult in some contexts, but the cost of acting out aggressively could be much higher than you wish to pay. Walking away in order to move towards a life that is values based versus emotionally reactive is a useful strategic retreat in a very heated moment.

After getting centred, if you need or want to stay in the situation, you can choose to ask directly for what is needed in the moment in a way that is both assertive and respectful to yourself and others involved. Compassionate assertiveness means speaking up for what will be helpful in the situation, for yourself, and for others when possible.

Another helpful action can be to choose forgiveness and letting go. Such a compassion-based response can help release steam during a tense moment, reducing suffering in the process. When my father taught me to drive, he also taught me intolerance of other drivers. For example, he showed me how to verbally and non-verbally curse and rage at a driver who cut our car off in traffic. As I got a bit older, I realized that those road rage moments were painful and prolonged, as my thoughts would ruminate on 'the jerk in the other car' throughout the rest of my day.

Eventually, I decided to try a different strategy. When in an angry motor vehicle moment, I began to use compassionate awareness to get off autopilot and compassionate acceptance of my own feelings and the imperfection of all humans in order to ease my struggle. Then I would try to take more values-based action. I would bring curiosity towards the other driver. Something in their life had brought them to the point of cutting me off in traffic. Perhaps they were suffering — maybe they were rushing to meet a sick family member in the hospital. Or maybe there was some other urgent reason for their behaviour. Regardless, I aim to shift my perspective to see them as a fellow human being who has their own traumas and tribulations in life, like the rest of us. If they live long enough they will experience the illness and deaths of friends and family and inevitably their bodies will break down and they will perish. Then from a compassionate mindset I wish them well with their challenges in life. I experienced that bringing even a small amount of compassion towards the person I am experiencing anger towards can be like a soothing balm to a deep ache. Then, the anger runs its course more quickly and my thoughts are freed up to focus on more valued topics.

Despair freakouts: When you feel like you just can't take it any more

It bears repeating: sometimes human life is very difficult. The pain we can experience in our bodies and deep within our minds can feel excruciating. In those moments our threat system will explore many options in trying to bring an end to this pain. Unfortunately, sometimes our minds will tell us that the way to end the pain is to end our life. In 2019, approximately one in ten high school students reported that they had attempted suicide over the previous twelve months.[6]

If you have suicidal thoughts, you are not alone. In a very distressing way, your mind is trying to help you find a solution to the pain. It is just not offering a flexible range of options at the moment.

When autopilot takes control

When hooked by suicidal thoughts and feelings you might catch yourself stuck with your mind ruminating and your body resisting moving towards what is good and meaningful in your life, such as exercise, spending time with friends and family, being out in nature and so on. In a particularly dark moment, some people become fused with their hopeless thoughts and begin to generate concrete, deadly plans.

Helpful action

If you find yourself in a moment of seriously contemplating ending your life (for example, making concrete plans), this is a sign that it is time to take valued and self-compassionate action. In this case it will most likely mean reaching out to supportive friends and family, contacting a mental health professional, calling a crisis line (such as Lifeline, Australia on 13 11 14, Lifeline Aotearoa's suicide crisis helpline on 0508 828 865, or 988 in the United States) or seeking urgent or emergency services at your local hospital or clinic. Autopilot means acting on short-term thinking, while Best Self action involves thinking in the long-term, even when it feels difficult.

If you are at a point where you feel like you can't go on, do not keep it a secret. Reach out for help right now. Safeguarding your life in the face of pain is both self-compassionate (as you care for yourself), and other-compassionate (as you continue living so you can make a positive difference in the lives of friends, family and others, who also each know suffering).

The power of '… and'

There are an infinite number of things people can freak out about. And most of us will experience moments of intense emotional distress at some points in life, often quite unexpectedly. We try to live the best lives we can and then, inevitably, something unfortunate happens that rocks our sense of safety and wellbeing. The writer Russ Harris calls this the 'reality slap.'[7] For example:

- being diagnosed with a serious illness
- being the victim of crime
- experiencing discrimination
- losing your job
- the death of someone you love
- your spouse filing for divorce.

All these situations come with very distressing emotions. Anxiety makes you want to run and hide. Anger makes you want to charge into a fight. And sadness may make you want to surrender to hopelessness. These are painful emotions to face, yet fighting those feelings often brings even more pain. Letting those emotions drive your behaviours runs the risk that they drive you away from behaving like the person you want to be.

Best Self action means accepting that human life can be very difficult *and* … The 'and' is the key. You can validate your experience of pain and then pivot towards valued and compassionate behaviour.

- **Getting diagnosed with kidney disease feels awful *and* I will take steps to maximize my health.**
- **Losing my job is so painful *and* I will treat myself with**

extra compassion while I look for a new one.
- My loved one has died. I feel emotionally devastated *and* I will give myself permission to grieve *and* I will reach out to a good friend *and* join a support group.
- That driver just cut me off on the highway. I feel rage and a desire to get revenge *and* acting on that is not who I want to be. I will slow my breathing down, let the anger pass, *and* I will let life be the teacher of that other driver — not me.

On top of that, there are highly distressing things happening all around us. Just turn on the news and see the stark reality of climate change, racism and social injustice, and a world that seems to be deeply divided by political ideology. It is not a matter of whether we will experience intense levels of distress, but of responding to the painful emotions and thoughts in a way that eases long-term suffering *and* moves us closer to values-based living, rather than emotion-driven reacting.

KEY POINTS

- In each distressing moment is potential for growth.

- You can use these moments to teach your threat system that the situation is tolerable, though unpleasant.

- Each unpleasant moment is an opportunity to hone your coping skills.

- In many cases you can teach your threat system that the situation is safe, though unpleasant – leading to less distress in the future.

PART 4

OVERCOMING CHALLENGES TO ACTING WITH COMPASSION

14

FEARS, BLOCKS AND RESISTANCES TO COMPASSION

Compassion has always been a defining feature of humanity. We survive because of our ability to cooperate and provide and receive protection and assistance. Because this is our nature, we feel safer (and therefore calmer) among people who care for our wellbeing and are motivated to ease or prevent our suffering.

Although compassion is connected with so many benefits, some people find it difficult to experience compassion, even when they try. Some feel repulsed by the idea of compassion for themselves, others, or both. Yet others even, initially, find the experience of compassion to be a highly distressing experience. The presence of such fears, blocks and resistances to compassion and all its benefits is what led Paul Gilbert to create Compassion Focused Therapy.

THE MINDFUL FREAK-OUT

What creates fears, blocks and resistances to compassion?

People who have been the victims of abuse by those who were supposed to care for and protect them (such as family, caregivers, close friends or romantic partners) can learn to associate caring with threat. Imagine the young child who has a caring parent who occasionally drinks too much and returns home to abuse them. They learn that caring equals danger. To feel safer they might push away from people or experiences that might open them up to compassion. They don't trust it. Even if they want to experience the benefits of compassion, whether from another person or working to bring compassion to themselves, they might find that doing so leads to the unwanted emergence of traumatic memories and the painful feelings they bring.

Other people might be blocked from experiencing compassion for other reasons. Perhaps they are open to compassion, but just don't know how to move towards it. Others could feel blocked because of life stressors interfering with their ability to experience compassion. For example, I have worked with a number of healthcare providers who experienced compassion fatigue during the early stages of the Covid pandemic. Caring for unprecedented volumes of severely ill and dying patients during a time of confusion regarding helpful medical interventions took a toll on their ability to care for the suffering of patients they faced day after day.

Some people are resistant to the idea of compassion. They might think compassion is synonymous with weakness or indulgence. Or they believe that only by being self-critical can they be successful with their goals.

There is another subset of people who are resistant to the idea of compassion because they grew up without experiencing it. They didn't have the experience of someone picking them up and speaking warmly to them when they scraped their knees as a toddler. They didn't have anyone in their life who cared. For them, compassion makes no sense. It is a foreign concept to them. As I write this, I recall my time working at a children's mental health clinic in Boston. I worked with some kids who were abused or neglected by their parents, placed into foster care only to receive similar treatment by their foster parents. It was one of the saddest experiences in my life to witness children who grow up without ever experiencing genuine compassion from a caregiver.

Working with your own fears, blocks or resistances to compassion

In spite of these fears, blocks and resistances to compassion, it is beneficial to build a compassionate mind so you can have access to one of the most helpful tools we humans have for easing or preventing suffering.

Let's now look at a variety of strategies that have been suggested by CFT therapists and researchers for fostering compassion in a person whose instinct tells them to stay away.[1]

Addressing misconceptions that compassion is weak or indulgent
Is compassion 'weak'?

Remember, compassion is not a feeling, it is a motive to ease or prevent suffering that you become aware of. Imagine someone is hurting your loved one — you walk in and notice their suffering. Would that elicit a weak response from you? Likely, you would do whatever it takes to help them.

How about police officers who serve and protect (a compassionate endeavour) by running towards the gunman in order to save lives when the shooting starts. Or how about firefighters rushing into a fiery building to rescue someone who is trapped. That is compassion in action.

Compassion is a powerful source of strength. Or how about the people around the world who get themselves out of bed and off to a job that is punishing to their body (and perhaps the spirit) so they can feed their children and prevent their suffering from hunger?

Is compassion weak? Not by any reasonable definition of the word.

Well, if it is not weak, is compassion indulgent?

Some people think of compassion as just doing things that feel good for you or others. Let's challenge that misconception.

Imagine your best friend calls and tells you they have been diagnosed with a life-threatening illness. They tell you that there is a treatment that is 99 percent effective, but it involves having surgery and they are phobic of needles and anaesthesia. You care deeply for this person. Would you indulge them by saying, 'Well, if that's how you feel then I support you'? Or would you try everything in your power to convince them to have the surgery and offer to be there to help out in any way you can?

If you had a six-year-old child who came to you and said, 'School is no fun. I want to sleep in and watch TV every day instead. And by the way, instead of vegetables, would you kindly give me cake and ice cream for every meal? Please — that would be so compassionate of you!' No, you wouldn't. What a life of suffering you would be setting this child up for if you indulged their every whim. It is compassionate to persuade them to go to school, eat their vegetables and do their homework because that sets them up for a future with less suffering.

Being overly indulgent is not compassionate, as it promotes greater suffering at a later time.

Dealing with the thought that you don't deserve compassion
Maybe you agree that compassion is a good thing to strive for — for other people. However, when it comes to compassion for yourself, you decline to accept it because you believe you are unworthy. Perhaps you have done something you regret and now believe you no longer deserve to receive compassion from others or yourself.

> *CFT emphasizes the wisdom of non-blame. While being compassionate doesn't mean we let ourselves off the hook for the mistakes we have made, it does recognize that even though we are responsible for our actions, we were driven largely by factors that were not our fault. It means that much of what led us to making those mistakes came about by factors outside our control. In fact, the person we grow into is shaped by factors we don't control. People do the best they can with how life, genes and evolution have moulded them.*

The question then is, what will help us make the best out of whatever life has brought our way? Try this thought experiment. Think about what it is about you that makes you feel unworthy of compassion. Now imagine that whatever it is was not your experience, but that of a specific person you care deeply about. Now they are the ones who feel unworthy of compassion. Would you write *them* off as being completely unworthy of compassion? Would you speak to them in the same way you speak to yourself about this? Most likely you would offer them more grace than you have offered yourself. You would likely be less harsh in your evaluation of this person. You'd be able to see the extenuating circumstances in their life — the things that led to their behaviour, which was shaped by an upbringing they did not choose.

You can then begin to bring that wiser, broader perspective to your own life.

Unhooking from the thought that you need to be hard on yourself to function at your best

Some people are convinced they will only achieve their goals in life if they default to a punishing, harsh, critical inner tone whenever they are imperfect or make a mistake. If this describes you, let's try another thought experiment adapted from Paul Gilbert's work on CFT.

Imagine you have a child who is a few years old and ready to start preschool. So, being the good parent that you are, you check out the local preschools to handpick which one you think will be best for your child's development. There are two local preschools to choose from.

The first school you go to visit is called The Tyrannical Academy. You are greeted by a frowning headmaster who says with casual disdain: 'We are a no-nonsense school. We do not tolerate mistakes. If your child makes a mistake, we shall criticize them sternly until they learn. Kindness is for losers. Now … give me your child and let me mould them!'

You let Headmaster Ratched know that you have another school to check out before making your decision and move on to the second preschool in your neighbourhood. This one is called The Compassionate Minds Academy. Here, you are greeted with a warm smile from the headmaster of that school, who explains, 'In our school, we strive to provide a nurturing experience for your child. When your child makes a mistake, we see that as an opportunity for learning and growth and we will help your child see how they can do things differently in the future.

We will help them to learn from their mistakes without punishing or shaming them.'

Assuming you want to choose the school that you believe will best nurture your child's development in the most effective ways, which school would you select? If you chose the compassionate approach for your child, perhaps you might be willing to sample such an approach for yourself.

Making sense of compassion when you have not experienced it from others

You can build up your compassion skills like any other skill — through practice. Think of all the things you routinely do that at some point seemed unfamiliar or outside your grasp. It is okay to start small to get a feel for it and then build your compassion muscles up over time. Try each of the compassionate mind practices in the book and see which one clicks for you, even a little. You might find it easier to focus on compassion for others at first, then gradually include accepting compassion from others and then offering it to yourself.

Facing a fear of compassion

You can treat a fear of compassion like you would any fear. If you begin to move towards it, facing the fear, you are much more likely to make progress with feeling safe using compassion than if you avoid it altogether. It is okay to start with small steps and work up at your own pace.

CFT researcher Dr Russel Kolts encourages people who fear compassion not to force it. He uses the example of frozen prawns, or shrimp. If you try to force thaw the prawns under running water, they will absorb water and get mushy and gross. Instead, allow them to defrost in the refrigerator naturally — it is worth the wait.[2]

When compassion is very anxiety triggering, you can start gently with basic mindfulness and soothing rhythm breathing to build up your grounding skills. Then you can ease into compassion using safe place imagery (see p. 99). From there, you might find it is easier to practise compassion for others, especially those you care about. Then, perhaps, move towards allowing yourself to be open to receiving caring from others (even from a pet) before you progress to giving yourself compassion. If some days a particular approach seems overwhelming, go back to earlier, easier practices.

> *Josiah is a 22-year-old self-described 'loner'. He is struggling socially and in trying to find a career path. He is lonely but feels intensely mistrusting of other people. Those rare times when people reach out to him bring out suspicion and irritability, which pushes people away. He would like to connect with others, but it feels unsafe. Josiah stays in the confines of his room for most of the day and avoids his parents, who only have unkind words and hostile tones for him. But the person with the most unkind hostility towards him is himself. He has hated himself for most of his life, having absorbed the emotional abuse from his parents for so many years.*
>
> *After becoming deeply depressed he began seeing a therapist for the first time. He used his therapy time to vent about how awful he and other people are, doing what he could to hold the therapy relationship at arm's length, terrified to feel vulnerable by really opening up to a compassionate presence. His fear of compassion blocked his progress until he agreed*

with his therapist's suggestion to get a pet. He picked out a cute little kitten that adored him. Taking care of this cat began to thaw his reluctance to feel compassion. That's when a compassionate life began to slowly open up to him.

KEY POINTS

- Compassion is strong, not weak.

- Compassion is not indulgent — it involves facing discomfort when it eases long-term suffering.

- You are worthy of compassion, even if you don't feel like you are.

- You can build your compassion muscles with practice and persistence, even if it feels scary.

15

WHEN THINGS DON'T GO WELL

In a moment of emotional distress anyone can be hijacked by their threat system and behave in a way they later regret. When this happens, it is quite tempting to resort to harsh self-criticism. Too often, people believe that punishing when they make a mistake is the most helpful reaction to have. Many people are raised and educated in environments that punish mistakes. It is ingrained in our educational systems: make a mistake and your grade is lowered. Make enough and you get an 'F' for 'failure'.

This might lead one to fuse with the notion that self-punishment is desirable. This can make people reluctant to give up their habit of harsh self-criticism when they make a mistake. People may have a fantasy that there's a way to achieve perfection in their lives. It can be tempting to believe that if they are hard on themselves, they will get to a point where they finally stop making mistakes.

What an enticing, yet utterly impossible fantasy. We are only human

THE MINDFUL FREAK-OUT

and all humans are imperfect and make mistakes. Therefore, despite our best intentions every one of us will continue to make mistakes.

> *Lynn gets incredibly jealous and suspicious of her boyfriend's intentions around other women. After all, she's been burnt before – twice! In those past relationships, her boyfriends cheated on her, leaving her alone and traumatized. Years have passed and she is in a new relationship, and it's going really well. She could see herself marrying this person and has never been so much in love.*
>
> *But her threat system never forgets what happened to her in the past. When her boyfriend goes out with friends, her mind torments her with images of him sleeping around. When she goes with him downtown, it tells her that he is checking out all the attractive women they pass, looking for a replacement for her. When this happens her threat system floods her with stress hormones, making her feel dread and rage towards her boyfriend. Many times, in a frenzied moment, she has confronted him, attacked his character and threatened to end their relationship. He responds with confusion and, over time, growing defensiveness.*
>
> *When things cool down, she realizes that she has overreacted. Fearing that she will sabotage her relationship, she seeks counselling to work through her relationship trauma from the past. When triggered, she now tries to slow things down and look at the situation, and her boyfriend, with greater compassion. It's working! When the thoughts and images of him cheating arise, she is able to understand why her threat system is on high alert*

and then she unhooks from the unhelpful thoughts. Their relationship has been growing deeper and more rewarding.

Recently, he was working late while she sat at home waiting for him. She flipped on the TV and, as bad luck would have it, the plot in that week's episode of her favourite show featured the main character being cheated on by her boyfriend. Lynn then looked at her watch and realized that he was supposed to be home 15 minutes earlier! She paced her living room, imagining the worst. When he came home, she greeted him by loudly demanding, 'Where the hell have you been!' This sparked a huge fight and a sleepless night for both.

She had been doing so well!

For most of us, that urge to punish ourselves with inner verbal abuse is tempting to say the least. But why do we do it and is it helpful?

Kristen Neff theorizes that self-criticism is a primitive social safety behaviour designed to make us self-punish for a perceived transgression rather than waiting to be punished by others.[1] By rushing to criticize ourselves, we are attempting to appease dominant detractors who may then reward our submissiveness by not kicking us out of the tribe and perhaps taking pity on us and offering to toss some scraps our way.

Even though we may have an instinct that tells us to be hard on ourselves when we make a mistake, not all instincts are helpful. For example, my instinct to dig into the leftover chocolate eclairs in the refrigerator rather than write this sentence is not helpful to me at the moment.

Giving in to the instinct to punish yourself for making a mistake comes at a cost. First of all, self-criticism serves to further activate your threat system, activating threat emotions and their unpleasant chemical counterparts. On top of that, some studies show that punishment can lead to diminished performance on tasks compared with praise. For example, a teaching style that emphasizes punishing student misbehaviour is associated with a 30 percent lower focus among students compared with a teaching style that emphasizes praising positive student behaviours.[2]

Are you still reluctant to give up self-criticism?

Paul Gilbert suggests trying the following thought experiment. Imagine you went to a wizard who casts a spell on you, making self-criticism vanish from your life — forever. There'll be no self-criticism when you make a mistake, no self-criticism when you are cranky and pick a fight with your significant other, and absolutely no self-criticism when you over-indulge in your go-to vice.

When you imagine this, what types of feelings show up? What are your reservations regarding giving up self-criticism? Do you see how holding on to self-punishment might feel like a security blanket you feel averse to giving up?

Gilbert suggests asking yourself the following questions:

- What does the self-critical part of you look like in your imagination?
- Notice your critic. What is it saying to you and how is it saying it?
- What does your critic feel about you?

Notice that the critic is usually saying some very nasty things to you — things you wouldn't dream of saying to another person. 'You are lazy, worthless, a jerk, can't do anything right.' Notice that the critic is angry and contemptuous of you. Notice whether your inner critic makes you feel motivated or demoralized. Is that really serving you well?

Shame-based self-criticism versus compassionate self-correction

Perhaps in a highly distressing moment, your autopilot took over and led you to treat someone you care about in a way that was hurtful. Or perhaps you impulsively let your anxiety talk you out of doing something that was important to you. When this happens you may be tempted to run towards the harsh reprimands of your inner critic: 'I'm a bad person for how I treated my partner!', 'I'm such a hopeless, weak person!' This can lead to feeling shame.

CFT distinguishes between shame-based self-criticism and compassionate self-correction. Shame-based self-criticism is steeped in threat emotions — a person regrets that they did something and has an urge to punish and condemn themselves. This is usually associated with a global evaluation of oneself. They feel their actions say something about them as a whole (e.g. 'I am bad'). It focuses on their past mistakes — and on rubbing their nose in it. And shame-based self-attacking can make a person want to withdraw, to crawl into a hole and disappear ('I am inferior to others').

After her over-reaction led to the big fight with her boyfriend, Lynn sank into self-loathing. 'I'm a lost cause,' she tells herself.

THE MINDFUL FREAK-OUT

> 'He's probably better off with another woman — I'm broken! Why would anyone want to be with me when I'll never be able to be like a normal girlfriend? I don't even know why I try when I'm just hopeless.' She wanted to text her boyfriend to apologize, but got stuck on the thought, 'I don't deserve forgiveness'. She kept her distance from her boyfriend for the next few nights, sleeping alone, snuggled uncomfortably with shame and despair.

Compassionate self-correction is different. It is open to a person's limitations and mistakes (as all humans have them), but with a focus on a desire to learn and grow. While a person might regret their actions that led to an undesired outcome, that regret is focused on a specific event ('I made a mistake'), rather than being a global negative judgment of themselves ('I'm broken'). Compassionate self-correction is forward-looking, with a focus on repairing the situation, atoning for a transgression and learning from a mistake. Rather than a hostile inner tone, self-correction is based on kindness and encouragement — and the wisdom to understand that people cannot possibly be anything other than imperfect, but we *can* try to learn from our mistakes.

> Lynn feels guilty that she exploded on her boyfriend, who had done nothing wrong. Yet she reminds herself that given what she has been through, it makes sense that she would have the impulse to behave this way. And, she tells herself, she had been making progress. She is working hard on her traumatic past in therapy and she had gone a long time without autopilot taking over when triggered. She reminds herself that she can't change

the past, but she can discuss this recent incident with her therapist, apologize to her boyfriend, and increase her daily mindfulness practice. Also, she'll set a goal to do a compassion exercise when her boyfriend is running late to help balance out the threat she feels. This was a regrettable lapse, but she is committed to learning and growing from it.

SKILL BUILDING:
COMPASSIONATE SELF-CORRECTION

Practise the following when an emotionally charged moment does not go well and you feel pulled towards self-criticism.

- Direct your focus on your five senses as you come back to the moment and prepare to turn inward.
- Allow your eyes to close or stare at a neutral spot in the room. Shift your focus to your soothing rhythm breathing for a couple of minutes to further centre yourself.
- Now, using one of the compassionate mind training approaches from Chapter 7, engage your compassionate mind. Think about embodying the elements of inner strength, wisdom and a commitment to being caring.
- Bring to mind the situation that did not go as well as you would have liked — perhaps a mistake you made or a behaviour you regret.
- From your compassionate mindset, view this experience as an opportunity to learn and grow. Using the benefit of greater wisdom and hindsight, is there a way you can

repair any consequences from this situation? What can you do to decrease the likelihood of a similar outcome in the future?

If you like to write or journal, another useful approach is compassionate letter writing. This involves writing yourself a letter from the perspective of your ideal compassionate other or from your compassionate mindset. This letter reflects an understanding of the complexities that led to the situation in question. It is 100 percent understanding and supportive.

Here are some general guidelines for compassionate letter writing:

- Start with soothing rhythm breathing to settle into the experience.
- Using an exercise from Chapter 7, engage your compassionate mind.
- Write a letter to yourself from the perspective of your compassionate self or ideal compassionate other.
- Use your compassionate mindset to avoid being perfectionistic about this exercise.
- 'Step back' and consider why the situation in question is difficult or painful for you. In the letter, empathetically validate the pain you feel about this situation (e.g. 'The emotional pain you feel is understandable given …').
- Be careful not to slip into criticizing (e.g. 'You always do this').
- Write as if you are committed to showing caring and support in order to help you live your best life.
- From this place of greater wisdom and caring, perhaps

offer a helpful (and nonjudgmental) suggestion for similar situations in the future. This would be the type of suggestion you would make to a close friend or loved one if they were in this situation.
- If a letter feels overwhelming to write, feel free to modify this to be a quick compassionate email or text.

Here's a sample letter:

Dear Lynn,

I can see that you are suffering right now — this is a difficult moment given how hard you have been working and how much your relationship means to you. It is very scary to have thoughts that you'll lose this relationship. I know that this regret you feel is so painful, that sometimes you want to give up.

This feels terrible right now, but remember that you have been working hard on this and have made wonderful progress. You are human and humans are imperfect and have powerful threat systems that can suddenly kick in and take us over — leading us to reacting in ways we later feel bad about. Given this, it makes sense that despite your best efforts, your threat system took over (though remember, it has been a while since it happened; your efforts are making a huge difference).

Remember, you are not alone in this. You have caring and supportive friends and family and it is okay to lean on them for support, just like you are always there for them. Also, you can take care of yourself, using the compassion work you have been practising. And you can learn from this situation, perhaps adding some more mindfulness practice into your daily routine to help recognize when autopilot is trying to take over.

Sincerely,

Lynn

Now, from a compassionate mindset, I invite you to write yourself a compassionate letter that addresses a mistake or imperfection that you notice your inner critic has been yelling at you about. You can keep it 'on file' to pull out and review when you are getting down on yourself. The goal of responding to a lapse or mistake is to pick yourself back up, learn from the experience, and make amends if needed.

KEY POINTS

- Humans are imperfect — we will make mistakes.
- We are often taught and take to heart that we need to be punished to learn from a mistake.
- Shame-based self-criticism is demoralizing.
- Compassionate self-correction aims to learn from mistakes — it is inspiring rather than demoralizing.

Beyond freaking out

In this book you have learned skills to help you get past very emotionally distressing moments in a way that minimizes suffering and facilitates values-based responding. However, the main strategies of compassionate awareness, compassionate acceptance and compassionate action do not have to be limited to only highly painful times. They can be useful for day-to-day life.

Being more aware of when you are beginning to feel annoyed, anxious, sad or even tired or hungry gives you useful information that can then be acted upon in a caring way. If we are not aware, we can mindlessly go through our days with less regard for our wellbeing (and possibly the wellbeing of those around us). Being more mindfully aware of what brings you joy, satisfaction, or an easing of suffering gives you the knowledge of what is needed to live a happier life.

Switching your automatic default from 'If it feels bad, fight or flee from it' (which we know throws gasoline on the suffering fire) to a more compassionate default can give a helpful boost to your inner strength and wisdom, which is needed to turn and effectively face challenges. Then you can choose values-based responding to those moments when you may not be highly distressed, but would still like to live your life in a way you feel good about.

And about values-based responding: this is not just how you want to be when things get tough. It is much broader than that. Values are indicators of how you want to live your life, the freak-out times and the joyful times and everywhere in between. Ideally, values answer the question of what you are going to do now. Not only now, as you complete this book, but every now that comes later.

This final sentiment is aspirational.

We have discussed compassion during difficult moments, but what if it wasn't confined to that — or to you and me? Imagine a world where compassion is taught in the same way as we teach children how to read and write, as a fundamental life skill. Imagine we spread the word about how our new brain and old brain can be cultivated with compassion to bring out the better angels of our nature. We humans can be a cruel and destructive species *and* we can be creative, generous and caring. If compassion was to take off as a global movement, just think how we could make the world better than the wars, racism and oppression that are the direct result of a lack of compassion. We have the technology and resources to feed the multitudes of children who go hungry around the world every day. We just, as of yet, don't have the collective compassion needed to do so. With the training of our minds to be more compassionate, the world could be a much better place.

At the very least we can start with ourselves and how we respond to the people and challenges around us.

Appendix 1

THE EMOTIONALLY DISTRESSING MOMENT RESCUE EXERCISE

This exercise pulls together a range of CFT and ACT approaches discussed in the book into one exercise that you can pull out and use when experiencing a highly distressing moment.

You are likely feeling a very intense emotion right now. Your threat system is trying to help you by pushing you to react impulsively; let's see if you can buy yourself some time to re-centre.

Begin to slow things down and notice that there is a struggle in your mind and body.

Pay attention to what your inner tone is like right now. Is it harsh, loud or judgmental? Try to shift to a tone of caring and gentleness towards yourself. If you were guiding a loved one through this difficult moment instead of yourself, how would your tone be? Wouldn't you try to be kind and helpful? Bring that to yourself now. Some people find placing a hand supportively over their heart can help set a more compassionate inner tone. Acknowledge that this is a moment of suffering and recognize that everyone suffers at times and you are not alone in this. Can you commit to trying to respond to this painful moment in a

THE MINDFUL FREAK-OUT

helpful way?

You might notice that your mind is warning you of what might happen at some time in the future, or it might bring you memories of something that happened in the past. See if you can come back to the present moment by focusing on your senses.

Notice your feet on the ground. If you are seated, observe what it feels like to gently but firmly push your feet down into the ground. Notice the texture of what you are standing on, sitting on or lying on. What does the furniture or floor feel like: is it soft or firm? Notice what the clothes on your body feel like. Notice the temperature in the air.

Notice what you can see around you. Notice people and objects. Notice the variety of textures, colours and sizes. Notice some things are moving and some things stay in place. See if you can notice one thing that you have never noticed before. It could be a big thing, like a person or painting, or it can be tiny, like the unique pattern or texture on your hand or an everyday object.

Notice sounds around you. What sounds can you hear that are nearby? And what sounds can you hear that are further away? Can you notice the sound of your own breathing? Notice what it sounds like when you deeply inhale. Now notice what it sounds like when you slowly exhale.

Notice your breath going in and out. Invite the fresh inhalation of air to flow down into your abdomen. Then follow the exhalation from your abdomen up and then out of your mouth or nose. Now invite your breath to deepen and slow. If it is comfortable for you, allow your exhalation to release even more slowly. As you exhale, allow yourself to let go of any struggle against your emotions that you become aware of. Try to find a slow and steady rhythm to your breath. Perhaps count to five as you inhale, hold your breath for one second, and exhale to a count of

Appendix 1

five or more. When your mind wanders away from your breath, remember this is what minds do and then gently direct it back to the rhythmic breathing. Allow yourself to take at least ten breaths this way.

Now, bring to mind a time when you were compassionate with another person or animal, a time you had a desire and commitment to being helpful. You had a sense of inner strength and the wisdom to not judge or blame. You were focused on easing suffering.

Revisit that time in your mind — seeing what you saw, hearing what you heard, and feeling what you felt. Now allow yourself to shift your body into a posture that represents that sense of inner strength, wisdom and caring. Allow yourself to have a compassionate facial expression, like a gentle smile you might have when greeting a friend. Bring the qualities of compassion with you as you face your current suffering.

From this more compassionate mindset, turn towards the uncomfortable emotions that have shown up for you. As you do so, the goal is to notice and let go of struggling or fighting with the emotions that might be happening automatically. Let's notice where in your body you are bracing or tightening against the emotions. You can begin by paying attention to your feet and notice if they are tensing, struggling or fidgeting. If so, invite your feet to soften as much as they are willing. We are not trying to relax our emotions away. Instead, let's see how much of the tensing, fighting and struggling we can let go of. Notice your calves, knees and upper legs. Let go of tensing or struggling there, as much as your body will allow. Notice your stomach muscles and see if they are squeezing. If so, invite them to soften. Same thing in your lower back. Notice tensing, struggling or fidgeting in your fingers, hands, wrists and forearms. Invite that tension to ease. Notice your upper arms, upper back and chest. Allow them to let go of the fight, as much as they are willing. Make space to hold the emotions as gently as you can. Now notice your neck, jaw and the space around your eyes and forehead. Allow them to let go of the struggle to resist the emotions as much as they are willing. Notice how different it can feel to meet painful emotions with compassionate willingness.

Now let's shift attention towards the threat-driven thoughts running through your mind. From that compassionate perspective sit back from these thoughts and watch them come and go. When you spot an unhelpful threat-based thought, notice that your mind is creating that thought and let it go. It doesn't mean you are trying to get rid of any thoughts, but instead you are trying to unhook from them.

It can help to bring to mind an image of sitting on the bank of a stream on a beautiful autumn day. Allow the unhelpful threat-based thoughts to be written on leaves that are floating down the stream, coming and going in their own time. Imagine seeing the leaves (your thoughts) float on by. Notice that you don't have to jump into the water to fish the leaves out or analyze them — just let them float by in their own time.

Next, notice that your threat system is fuelling a number of urges. Notice and name the ones you are experiencing. For example, if you are feeling angry, you might notice the urge to lash out. If you are feeling anxious, you might have urges to avoid something or use safety behaviours. If you are feeling despair, you might notice an urge to retreat from your life.

Remember, these urges are messages sent by your threat system. You can choose whether to act on them or choose another action. If you were feeling your best and most compassionate, how would you want to act at this moment? Now see if you can commit to this action. Then, notice whether this moved your life in a more desirable direction than if you had acted on an impulsive threat-based urge or instinct.

It is okay to cycle through this exercise as much as you need during an emotional storm.

Appendix 2

EXERCISE RECORD FORM

Practise those exercises that build needed skills, and record your progress on this form.

If you are having difficulty with getting off autopilot these exercises can help:

COMPASSIONATE AWARENESS EXERCISES

Exercise	See page:	Dates completed	Notes/observations
Mindful pause	29		
Compassionate tone	34		

Appendix 2

Compassionate touch	35		
Soothing rhythm breathing	42		
Sensory awareness training	45		
Mindful awareness of emotions	48		
Being the noticer	53		
Incorporating present moment awareness into your daily routine	55		
Breathing out struggle	121		
Urge surfing	147		

THE MINDFUL FREAK-OUT

If you are having difficulty tolerating threat-based feelings or are hooked by threat-thoughts, these exercises can help:

COMPASSIONATE ACCEPTANCE EXERCISES

Exercise	See page:	Dates completed	Notes/observations
Compassionate colour	98		
Safe place imagery	99		
Metta (loving-kindness) meditation	100		
Compassionate memories: compassion flowing to you	102		
Compassionate memories: compassion flowing to another	103		

Appendix 2

Ideal compassionate other	104		
Ideal compassionate self	105		
Compassion for the freaked-out self	108		
Self-compassion using your image	109		
Compassionate behaviour practice (self and other)	110		
Mindful body scan	118		
Defusion from thoughts	129		
Compassionate self-correction	239		

THE MINDFUL FREAK-OUT

If you are having difficulty choosing how to respond to a highly distressing moment these exercises can help:

Taking Best Self action exercises

Exercises	See page:	Dates completed	Notes/observations
Mindful awareness of urges	144		
Values clarification: tombstone	156		
Values clarification: a well-lived life	157		
Values clarification: my final years	158		
Choosing your Best Self response	168		
Identifying immediate values-based behaviours	178		

Appendix 3

RESCUE STRATEGY FOR BEING AT YOUR BEST WHEN LIFE IS AT ITS WORST: **BRIEF OUTLINE**

01 COMPASSIONATE AWARENESS: GET OFF AUTOPILOT
   What helps:
   - Notice suffering and slow down.
   - Set an intention to do what is helpful.
   - Anchor in the present moment using breath and senses.

02 COMPASSIONATE ACCEPTANCE: COMPASSIONATELY FACE THE MOMENT
   What helps:
   - Engage compassionate mind.
   - Notice and release struggle.
   - Unhook from unhelpful thoughts.

03 COMPASSIONATE ACTION: RESPOND BASED ON YOUR BEST SELF
   What helps:
   - Notice and name your urge to react.
   - Choose your Best Self response.
   - Act and notice the outcome.

Acknowledgements

This book would not exist without the work Steven Hayes and Paul Gilbert put into developing ACT and CFT. Their work has helped ease the suffering of countless people across the planet. They have each taken timeless wisdom, made it accessible for the minds of today, and through research have proven what people have intuited for thousands of years: that mindfulness and compassion are powerful tools to make human life better.

As an anxiety disorder and OCD specialist, I have noticed that the focus in this community of researchers and practitioners has been on facing fears in order to alleviate a phobic problem. This is important, no doubt. However, one's suffering while facing a fear is, in my humble opinion, too often neglected. Russ Harris, however, writes about how ACT can be used to help people get through such difficult moments with less suffering. He advocates facing intense emotional moments using three steps: Acknowledging, Coming Back, and Engaging — his 'dropping anchor' concept. This was my initial inspiration for the concepts in this book. My goal was to infuse compassionate engagement throughout the dropping anchor practice and write a book to help people get better at dropping their anchors to ride out emotional storms in a way that addresses suffering while encouraging values-based responding.

I am deeply grateful for my friends and colleagues Ellen Pitrowski, Michael McGee and Kim Rockwell-Evans for their support and assistance with the manuscript. Thanks to Chris Fraser for the feedback and encouragement of my efforts to integrate CFT and ACT for the challenge of easing suffering during highly distressing moments. And a huge thank you to the team at Exisle Publishing, especially Anouska Jones, Gareth St John Thomas and Karen Gee for their consistent encouragement and the hard work and attention they have put into this book.

And none of this would have been possible without the support of my amazing wife and best friend Anya and our three inspiring children, Alex, Jessie and Lana. My soothing system is continuously bolstered by your presence in my life.

A final endless debt of gratitude goes to the organ donor whose gift of a kidney 20+ years ago was the purest act of compassion I have ever experienced. Every book I have written, client I have helped, child I have raised, and breath I have taken was made possible because of you.

Endnotes

Introduction
1. Merrian-Webster definition of 'freak-out', accessed 29 October 2022, www.merriam-webster.com/dictionary/freak-out.

2. Collins English Dictionary definition of 'freak-out', accessed 29 October 2022, www.collinsdictionary.com/us/dictionary/english/freak-out.

3. Kirby, J.N. 2017, 'Compassion interventions: The programmes, the evidence, and implications for research and practice', *Psychol Psychother Theory Res Pract*, 90(3), pp. 432–55, doi:10.1111/papt.12104.

4. Azizi, M., Sepehri, S., Demehri, F. 2021, 'Effect of acceptance and commitment therapy combined with compassion-focused therapy on behavioral problems and mother-child interactions in children with hearing impairment', *Audit Vestib Res*, 30(4), pp. 256–63, doi:10.18502/avr.v30i4.7473.

5. Tirch, D.D., Schoendorff, B., Silberstein, L.R. 2014, *The ACT Practitioner's Guide to the Science of Compassion: Tools for fostering psychological flexibility*, New Harbinger Publications, Oakland.

Chapter 3
1. Porges, S.W. 2007, 'The polyvagal perspective', *Biol Psychol*, 74(2), pp. 116–43, doi:10.1016/j.biopsycho.2006.06.009.

2. Neff, D.K. 2015, *Self-Compassion: The proven power of being kind to yourself*, William Morrow Paperbacks, New York.

Chapter 4
1. Kabat-Zinn, J. 2011, 'Some reflections on the origins of MBSR, skillful means, and the trouble with maps', *Contemp Buddhism*, 212(1),

pp. 281–306, doi:10.1080/14639947.2011.564844.

2. Hayes, S.C., Smith, S. 2005, *Get Out of Your Mind and Into Your Life: The new Acceptance and Commitment Therapy*, New Harbinger Publications, Oakland.

3. Steffen, P.R., Bartlett, D., Channell, R.M., et al. 2021, 'Integrating breathing techniques into psychotherapy to improve HRV: Which approach is best?' *Front Psychol*, 12, p. 624254, doi:10.3389/fpsyg.2021.624254.

4. Zaccaro, A., Piarulli, A., Laurino, M. et al. 2018, 'How breath-control can change your life: A systematic review on psychophysiological correlates of slow breathing', *Front Hum Neurosci*, 12, p. 353, doi:10.3389/fnhum.2018.00353.

5. Gilbert, P. 2014, 'The origins and nature of compassion focused therapy', *Br J Clin Psychol*, 53(1), pp. 6–41, doi:10.1111/bjc.12043.

6. Zhang, D., Lee, E.K.P., Mak, E.C.W., Ho, C.Y., Wong, S.Y.S. 2021, 'Mindfulness-based interventions: An overall review', *Br Med Bull*, published online 21 April, ldab005, doi:10.1093/bmb/ldab005.

Chapter 6

1. Kirby, J.N. 2017, 'Compassion interventions: The programmes, the evidence, and implications for research and practice', *Psychol Psychother Theory Res Pract*, 90(3), pp. 432–55, doi:10.1111/papt.12104; Kang, Y., Gray, J.R., Dovidio, J.F. 2014, 'The nondiscriminating heart: Lovingkindness meditation training decreases implicit intergroup bias', *J Exp Psychol Gen*, 143(3), pp. 1306–13, doi:10.1037/a0034150; Kim, J.J., Parker, S.L., Doty, J.R., Cunnington, R., Gilbert, P., Kirby, J.N. 2020, 'Neurophysiological and behavioural markers of compassion', *Sci Rep*, 10(1), p. 6789, doi:10.1038/s41598-020-63846-3; Kirby, J.N., Tellegen, C.L., Steindl, S.R. 2017, 'A meta-analysis of compassion-based interventions:

Current state of knowledge and future directions', *Behav Ther*, 48(6), pp. 778–92, doi:10.1016/j.beth.2017.06.003; Klimecki, O.M. 2015, 'The plasticity of social emotions', *Soc Neurosci*, 10(5), pp. 466–73, doi:10.10 80/17470919.2015.1087427; Klimecki, O.M. 2019, 'The role of empathy and compassion in conflict resolution', *Emot Rev*, 11(4), pp. 310–25, doi:10.1177/1754073919838609; MacBeth, A., Gumley, A. 2012, 'Exploring compassion: A meta-analysis of the association between self-compassion and psychopathology', *Clin Psychol Rev*, 32(6), pp. 545–52, doi:10.1016/j.cpr.2012.06.003; Matos, M., Duarte, C., Duarte, J., et al. 2017, 'Psychological and physiological effects of compassionate mind training: A pilot randomised controlled study', *Mindfulness*, 8(6), pp. 1699–712, doi:10.1007/s12671-017-0745-7; Zabelina D.L., Robinson, M.D. 2010, 'Don't be so hard on yourself: Self-compassion facilitates creative originality among self-judgmental individuals', *Creat Res J*, 22(3), pp. 288–93, doi:10.1080/10400419.2010.503538.

2. Leeb, R.T., Lewis, T., Zolotor, A.J. 2011, 'A review of physical and mental health consequences of child abuse and neglect and implications for practice', *Am J Lifestyle Med*, 5(5), pp. 454–68, doi:10.1177/1559827611410266.

3. Gilbert P. 2014.

4. Gilbert P. 2014.

5. Gilbert P. 2010, *The Compassionate Mind: A new approach to life's challenges*, Constable, London.

Chapter 7

1. Tirch, D.D., Schoendorff, B., Silberstein, L.R. 2014; Gilbert, P. 2014; Gilbert, P. 2010; Irons, C., Beaumont, E. 2017, *The Compassionate Mind Workbook: A step-by-step guide to developing your compassionate self*, Robinson, London.

2. Daly, A. 2020, 'Exploring the effects of metta meditation on

emotional regulation: Using semi structured interviews on adult novice meditators', The IIE, accessed 31 October 2022, http://iiespace.iie.ac.za/handle/11622/511; Frick, A., Thinnes, I., Stangier, U. 2020, 'Metta-based group meditation and individual cognitive behavioral therapy (MeCBT) for chronic depression: Study protocol for a randomized controlled trial', *Trials*, 21(1), p. 20, doi:10.1186/s13063-019-3815-4; Nilsson, H. 2016, 'Socioexistential mindfulness: Bringing empathy and compassion into health care practice', *Spiritual Clin Pract*, 3(1), pp. 22–31, doi:10.1037/scp0000092.

Chapter 8
1. Neff, D.K. 2015, p. 93.

2. Collins, M., Harris, R. 2009, 'The happiness trap', *J Happiness Stud*,10(4), pp. 497–8, doi:10.1007/s10902-009-9133-x.

Chapter 9
1. Wegner, D.M., Schneider, D.J., Carter, S.R., White, T.L. 1987, 'Paradoxical effects of thought suppression', *J Pers Soc Psychol*, 53, pp. 5–13, doi:10.1037/0022-3514.53.1.5.

2. Goodman, E. 2020, *Your Anxiety Beast and You: A compassionate guide to living in an increasingly anxious world*, Exisle Publishing, Dunedin.

Chapter 10
1. Marlatt, G.A., Gordon, J.R. 1985, *Relapse Prevention: Maintenance strategies in the treatment of addictive behaviors*, Guilford Press, London.

2. Abouzed. M., et al. 2020, 'Urge surfing intervention in patient with chronic atopic dermatitis', accessed 13 November 2022, www.azmj.eg.net/article.asp?issn=1687-1693;year=2020;volume=18;issue=4;spage=449;epage=452;aulast=Abouzed; Bowen, S., Marlatt, A. 2009, 'Surfing the urge: Brief mindfulness-based intervention for college

student smokers', *Psychol Addict Behav*, 23(4), pp. 666–71, doi:10.1037/a0017127; Ostafin, B.D., Marlatt, G.A. 2008, 'Surfing the urge: Experiential acceptance moderates the relation between automatic alcohol motivation and hazardous drinking', *J Soc Clin Psychol*, 27(4), pp. 404–18, doi:10.1521/jscp.2008.27.4.404.

Chapter 11

1. Hayes, S.C. 2019, *A Liberated Mind: How to pivot toward what matters*, Penguin Publishing Group, New York.

Chapter 12

1. Lundgren, T., Luoma, J.B., Dahl, J., Strosahl, K., Melin, L. 2012, 'The bull's-eye values survey: A psychometric evaluation', *Cogn Behav Pract*, 19(4), pp. 518–26, doi:10.1016/j.cbpra.2012.01.004.

2. Craske, M.G., Treanor, M., Conway, C., Zbozinek, T., Vervliet, B. 2014, 'Maximizing exposure therapy: An inhibitory learning approach', *Behav Res Ther*, 58, pp. 10–23. doi:10.1016/j.brat.2014.04.006.

Chapter 13

1. Wilhelm, F.H., Gevirtz, R., Roth, W.T. 2001, 'Respiratory dysregulation in anxiety, functional cardiac, and pain disorders: Assessment, phenomenology, and treatment', *Behav Modif*, 25(4), pp. 513–45, doi:10.1177/0145445501254003.

2. Meadows, D.G. 2014, *The Sleep Book: How to sleep well every night*, CreateSpace Independent Publishing Platform.

3. Esch, T., Stefano, G.B. 2011, 'The neurobiological link between compassion and love', *Med Sci Monit*, 17(3), pp. RA65–75, doi:10.12659/MSM.881441.

4. Trauer, J.M., Qian, M.Y., Doyle, J.S., Rajaratnam, S.M.W., Cunnington, D. 2015, 'Cognitive behavioral therapy for chronic insomnia', *Ann Intern Med*, 163(3), pp. 191–204, doi:10.7326/M14-2841.

5. Salari, N., Khazaie, H., Hosseinian-Far, A. et al. 2020, 'The effect of acceptance and commitment therapy on insomnia and sleep quality: A systematic review', *BMC Neurol*, 20(1), p. 300, doi:10.1186/s12883-020-01883-1.

6. Ivey-Stephenson, A.Z., Demissie, Z., Crosby, A.E., et al. 2019, 'Suicidal ideation and behaviors among high school students: Youth risk behavior survey, United States, 2019', *MMWR Morb Mortal Wkly Rep*, 69(1), pp. 47–55, doi:10.15585/mmwr.su6901a6.

7. Harris, R. 2012, *The Reality Slap: Finding peace and fulfillment when life hurts*, New Harbinger Publications, Oakland.

Chapter 14
1. Gilbert, P., McEwan, K., Matos, M., Rivis, A. 2011, 'Fears of compassion: Development of three self-report measures', *Psychol Psychother Theory Res Pract*, 84(3), pp. 239–55, doi:10.1348/147608310X526511; Steindl, S., Bell, T., Dixon, A., Kirby, J. 2022, 'Therapist perspectives on working with fears, blocks and resistances to compassion in compassion focused therapy', *Couns Psychother Res*, published online 29 March, doi:10.1002/capr.12530.

2. Kolts, R.L. 2016, *CFT Made Simple: A clinician's guide to practicing compassion-focused therapy*, New Harbinger Publications, Oakland.

Chapter 15
1. Neff, D.K. 2015, p. 24.

2. 'Praise, rather than punish, to see up to 30% greater focus in the classroom', ScienceDaily, accessed 29 October 2022, www.sciencedaily.com/releases/2020/01/200129091430.htm.

INDEX

A

abdominal breathing 42-4, 49
acceptance
  explained 61-2
  meaning 16
  see also compassionate acceptance
Acceptance and Commitment Therapy (ACT)
  about living your life 66-7
  acceptance of thoughts 125-6
  act of acceptance 64-5
  adding CFT 18-19
  defusion metaphors 130-6
  encourages mindfulness 41
  fear of flying 208
  overlapping strategies 15-17
  sensory experiencing 82
  workability concept 163-7
adversity
  advice to loved one 163
  responding to 160-1
  role-models for handling 161-2
AFGO (Another Freaking Growth Opportunity)
  day after night of insomnia 205
  explained 193
  fear of flying 208-9
  using difficult moments 192-3
alcohol, battle with 126-7
American Splendor (movie) 109-10
anchor in present moment 4, 39-58
'... and', power of 217-18
anger
  on autopilot 213
  compassionate 82
  controlling 213-15
  flaring up 212-13
  regretted later 212
animals

  no concept of death 87-8
  reactions to threats 85
anxiety, list of relief activities 176
anxiety beast metaphor 130-1
assertiveness, compassionate 214-15
attention, ability to focus 78
attention shifting exercise 96-7
autopilot
  ability to disengage 54
  disengaging 40, 173-4
  distressing moments 3-4
  existential panic 210
  during flight turbulence 207-8
  getting off 25-6, 255
  insomnia situations 202-3
  during panic attacks 196-7
  social anxiety situations 199-201
  suicidal thoughts 216
  when anger takes over 213
avoidance behaviours
  fear of flying 208
  trains threat system 196-7
  used to face fears 200
awareness *see* compassionate awareness

B

beach ball in the pool metaphor 134
befriending yourself 107-9
behaviour, compassionate 81, 110-13, 217-18
being the noticer exercise 53-4
Best Self
  choosing your responses 149-55, 168-71
  compassionate action 6-8
  compassionate behaviour 217-18
  describing 152
  martial arts champion 160
  perspective of 187-8

rescue strategy 255-6
taking action, exercise record form 254
blame, wisdom of non-blame 227-8
brain *see* human brain
breathing
   abdominal 42-4, 49
   different strategies 44
   5, 4, 3, 2, 1 method 46
   focus on 41-2
   mindful 4, 42
   rescue exercise 245-9
   soothing rhythm 42-4, 49
breathing out struggle exercise 121
Bruce, battle with alcohol 126-7
Buddha, awareness of approaching death 87-8
Bueller, Ferris 27

C

car accident, daughter's 11, 12, 13-15, 17-19
Carmelita, social anxiety 165-6
Caroline, suffers insomnia 201
challenging moments, responding to 187-8
compassion
   acts of, for others 111
   aspects decreased by 72
   aspects increased by 72
   benefits of cultivating 71-2
   deprivation of 74
   easing into 230-1
   explained 74-5
   facing fear of 229-31
   fears, blocks and resistance to 224-6
   feature of humanity 223
   feeling undeserving of 227-8
   for freaked-out self 108-9
   key religious concept 71
   learning from a pet 231
   main strategies 243-4
   making sense of 229
   misconceptions about 225-6
   of others 73-4
   vs punishment 228-9
   shifting attention towards 96-7
   source of 73-4
   strategies to foster 225-31
   teach as life skill 244
   three targets (flows) of 82-3
Compassion Focused Therapy (CFT)
   approach to insomnia 204
   Buddhist-informed definition 74-5
   building compassion 71-2
   emotions regulation 89-93
   explained 69
   fear of flying 208
   focus on compassion 18-19
   mindful breathing 41-2
   sensory experiencing 82
compassionate acceptance
   exercise record form 252-3
   painful moments 5-6
   rescue strategy 255
   see also acceptance
compassionate action, Best Self 6-8
compassionate awareness
   awareness strategies 15-16
   to compassionate acceptance 57
   exercise record form 250-1
compassionate behaviour 81, 110-13, 217-18
compassionate colour exercise 98-9
compassionate reasoning 80-1
compassionate self, acting like your ideal 105-7
compassionate tone
   to fuel helpful intent 33
   practising 34-5
compassionate touch
   for others 35
   self-touch 36
compassion-focused imagery 98-107
conflict
   avoiding 160

with a loved one 95–6
Covid prevention mask, causing rage 211
Craske, Dr Michelle 188

D
daily routine, awareness of 55–6
Dalai Lama, got angry 212
Darius, fear of panic attacks 166–7
death, humans' awareness of 87–8
defusion
    explained 16–17, 124
    metaphors 130–6
    from thoughts 129
despair freak-outs 215–16
distress, tolerance of 76
distressing moments *see* adversity
distressing thoughts, struggling with 62–3
drive system, overactive 91–2
driving, fear of 159–60

E
Eliza, no response to text 191
emotional distress, workability of avoiding 66–7
emotional pain, struggling against 179
emotional quicksand metaphor 116–17
emotions
    mindfully aware of 48–51
    threat-based 23–5
    tipping point 48
    see also painful emotions
empathy, explained 77
exercise record forms
    compassionate acceptance 252–3
    compassionate awareness 250–1
    taking Best Self action 254
exercises
    attention shifting 96–7
    being the noticer 53–4
    breathing out struggle 121
    compassionate colour 98–9

dealing with anxious thoughts 62–3
emotionally distressing moment rescue 245–9
ideal compassionate other 104–5
ideal compassionate self 105–7
mindful body scan 118–20
My Final Years values clarification 158–9
reflection on well-lived life 157–8
safe place imagery 99–100
tombstone 156–7
urge surfing 147–8
see also skill building
existential panic
    approaching death 209–11
    living with 'faith' 211
exposure therapy 197–8

F
'faith', difficulty embracing 210
family, value of 153
fears
    avoidant behaviours 200
    of compassion 229–31
    death and existential panic 209–11
    of driving 159
    of flying 163, 193, 208–9
    public speaking 70–1
    see also panic attacks
feelings, compassionate approach to 81–2
fight-or-flight response 3–4, 195–6
5, 4, 3, 2, 1 breathing method 46
flying
    fear of 163, 193
    flight turbulence 207–8
    helpful action options 208–9
freaking out, don't count on not 13–15
'freak-out', meaning 9–11
freak-outs, response to 11–13, 191–2
future, uncertain 39

THE MINDFUL FREAK-OUT

G
Giamatti, Paul 109–10
Gilbert, Dr Paul 69–70
  old brain/new brain 86
global pandemic, stress of 211
guard dog metaphor 131

H
Harris, Dr Russ 117, 217
Hayes, Steven 65
high school students, suicidal thoughts 215
Hot Potato (game) 213
human brain
  ancient parts 86
  old brain/new brain 86–7
humans survival strategy 73
hunters and gatherers, behaviour 198–9

I
imagery
  compassion-focused 98–107
  power of 79
insomnia
  acceptance of 203–6
  catastrophic thoughts 40
  feelings the day after 205–6
  middle-of-the-night freak-out 201–6
  taking mindful approach 204–5

J
John 80–1
Josiah, mistrusting of other people 230
Jung, Carl 115–16

K
Kabat-Zinn, Dr Jon 40
Kolts, Dr Russel 229

L
leaves on a stream simile 132
letter writing, to self 240–2

life review
  Final Years clarification exercise 158–9
  reflecting on life 157
  what would you change 163–4
Lifeline Aotearoa 216
Lifeline Australia 216
loving kindness meditation 91–2
Lynn
  sinks into self-loathing 237–8
  suspicious of boyfriend 234–5
  in therapy 238–9

M
'Make Me Angry' (game show) 213–14
Malik, man of rage 177
Meadows, Dr Guy 203–4
meditation, metta (loving-kindness) 100–2
memories, compassionate 102–4
memory
  access a compassionate mindset 104
  compassion flowing to another 103
  compassion flowing to you 102–3
metta meditation 100–2
mindful body scan 118–20
mindful pause 29–30
mindfulness
  acceptance of thoughts 125–6
  awareness of emotions 48–51
  awareness of urges 144–6
  breathing 41–2
  to disengage autopilot 40
  focus of attention 78
  present moment awareness 55–6
  present observations 40–1
  using body for awareness 47–8
mistakes, punishment in schools 228–9, 233
mortality, awareness of our own 157–9
My Final Years values clarification 158–9

N
nature defusion metaphors 131–3

Index

Neff, Dr Kristen 35, 116, 235
non-judgment, meaning of 76-7

O
observing mind
  explained 16
  self-as-context 52
  turning on 52-5
ocean waves metaphor 132-3
other people's children on the plane metaphor 134-5

P
pace of life, overly busy 27-8
painful emotions
  acceptance of struggle 62-4
  avoiding 61-2
  facing 6
painful moments, face with compassion 5-6
panic attacks
  avoidant strategies 196
  exposure therapy 197-8
  fear of 194-8
  helpful action 197-8
  managing 166-7, 175
  teachable moment 198
pausing, practise 29-30
Pekar, Harry 109-10
perfectionism trap, all-or-nothing 187
pet poodle, Sprinkles 85
pets, learning compassion from 231
Pope Francis, slapped woman's hand 154
power of '... and' 217-18
prawns, thawing 229-30
predator, sabre-toothed 90
preschool teacher, defusion strategy 135-6
present moment
  anchoring in 39-58
  contacting the 16
'psychological flexibility' 15
public speaking, fear of 70-1, 194

punishment
  vs compassion 231
  for making mistakes 233
  for mistakes in schools 228-9
  reducing student focus 236
punishment vs compassion 228-9

R
rage, regretted later 212
Raven, fear of panic attacks 175
'reality slap' 217
reasoning, compassionate 80-1
relationship trauma, from the past 234-5
religion, comforting refuge 210
rescue strategy, for being Best Self 255-6
road rage 214-15
Roy, angry at boss 144

S
sabre-toothed predator 90
sadness, compassionate 82
safe place imagery exercise 99-100
safety behaviours, fear of flying 208
Sasha, panics while driving 124
sea turtle, species survival 73
Sean, struggle to leave home 175
self-as-context see observing mind
self-compassion 107-9
  acts of 110-11
  the case for 83-8
  using your image 109-10
self-correction, compassionate 237-42
self-criticism
  on autopilot 28
  vs compassionate self-correction 237-9
  getting in first 235-6
  reluctant to give up 236-7
self-touch, compassionate 36
sensory awareness training 45-6
sensory experiencing 82
Shari, disagreement with spouse 164-5

269

THE MINDFUL FREAK-OUT

Silver Linings Playbook (movie) 173–4
skill building
  being the noticer 53–4
  breathing out struggle 121
  choosing Best Self response 168–71
  compassionate self-correction 239–42
  compassionate tone 34–5
  compassionate touch 35–6
  defusion from thoughts 129
  identifying values-based behaviours 178
  mindful awareness of emotions 48–51
  mindful awareness of urges 144–6
  mindful body scan 118–20
  mindful pause 29–30
  present moment awareness 55–6
  sensory awareness training 45–6
  soothing rhythm breathing 42–4
  urge surfing 147–8
  using body for mindful awareness 47–8
  values clarification–tombstone exercise 156–7
sleep
  lack of 201–6
  riddle about 201
sleep deprivation, feeling result of 205–6
social anxiety
  causing isolation 165–6
  in social spotlight 198–201
  struggle to leave home 175
social situations, 'quick fixes' 81
soothing rhythm breathing 42–4, 49
soothing/safeness system 92–3
statistics, suicidal thoughts, high school students 215
struggle switch metaphor 117–20
suffering
  alleviating and preventing 78–82
  engaging with 75–7
  sensitivity to 75
suicidal thoughts 215–16
suicide crisis helplines 216

Suyin, phobia of driving 159–60
sympathy, meaning of 75–6

T

temper, post-rage shame 177–8
'The Devil's bargain' talk 65–6
thoughts
  anxious 199–200
  awareness of 127–36
  context dependent 126–7
  dealing with anxiety 62–3
  as leaves on a stream 132
  mindful acceptance of 125–6
  unhelpful thoughts 179–80
    see also defusion
threat system
  function of 89–93
  hijacks you 90
  sees flying as dangerous 207–8
  training yours 193–4
threats
  emotional response to 23–5
  instinctive reaction to 31–2
  in the mind 88
  reactions to 84
thunderstorm metaphor 133
time machine, test driving 89–92
Tina, hates her job 128
toddler sheriff metaphor 131
tombstone exercise 156–7
touch *see* compassionate touch
traumatic experiences
  animal *vs* human reactions 85–6
  reliving 85–6
triggering situations, changing response to 180–2
turbulence
  freak-out moment 206–9
  as an opportunity 193

U

uncertainty
  action in the face of 211
    see also existential panic
uncomfortable feelings, squeezing out 63–4
unhelpful thoughts
  fused with 179–80
  unhooking from 6, 123–4
urge surfing, explained 146
urge to react, notice and name 7
urges
  explained 142–4
  mindful awareness of 144–6

V

values
  clarification 156–7
  defining yours 152–4
  not clarified 180
values-based action
  barriers to 179–84
  overcoming your barriers 184–6
  what happens after 188–9
values-based behaviours, identifying 178

W

waterfall metaphor 133
wellbeing, motivation to care for 76
white knuckling 115–16
Williams, Robin 162

Z

Zara, fear of flying 163
Zuri, fear of public speaking 70–1